# HERB
## CONTRAINDICATIONS
### AND
# DRUG
## INTERACTIONS

With Appendices
Addressing Specific
**CONDITIONS**
And
**MEDICINES**

Francis Brinker, N.D.

Eclectic Institute, Inc.
Sandy, Oregon

Combining herbal use with any prescribed medication
should only be done after consultation with a physician.
Information provided in this book is not intended to take
the place of instructions provided by one's doctor.

For information about permission to reproduce selections
from this book, write to:
Permissions
Eclectic Institute, Inc.
14385 S.E. Lusted Road
Sandy, Oregon 97055


Printed in the USA
ISBN 0-9659135-0-3   paperback
Library of Congress Catalog Card Number:   97-61558


Editorial and Production by Nancy Stodart
Book and Cover design by Richard Stodart
Composition by A. R. Eguiguren

# Contents

# Foreword

Recent years have seen an explosion of interest in botanical medicine, among both the general public and the medical profession. The results of clinical studies have proved beyond doubt that—to give but a few examples—garlic and ginkgo have an important role to play in the treatment of cardiovascular disease, and St. John's wort is effective for mild to moderate depression (thus confirming its traditional role as a 'nervine tonic'). There has been a recognition, in short, that herbal medicines have significant pharmacological activity.

With the recognition of benefit, however, comes that of risk, albeit slight. If phytotherapy is to play a meaningful role—as I believe it should—in health care in the twenty-first century, it is essential that physicians, pharmacists, and patients understand when certain herbs should not be used at therapeutic dosage—in pregnancy, in certain disease conditions, or in combination with specific pharmaceutical drugs. This book is intended to address the 'knowledge vacuum' that exists at present.

It must be acknowledged at the outset that some of the contraindications given here would not find ready agreement among all botanical practitioners. For example, choleretic and cholagogue herbs are considered by many phytotherapists (including myself) to be the mainstay of gallstone treatment, since they increase the solubility of cholesterol in bile. Both tradition and clinical practice bear witness to the effectiveness of this approach.

The fact that this manual proscribes such herbs for patients with gallstones is, however, more a reflection of the text's aims and scope than evidence of a lack of agreement on this issue. For the treatment of serious medical problems should be undertaken by qualified practitioners, and should not be the subject of self-medication. Texts addressed to the general public, therefore, or even to professionals whose knowledge of a particular area is scanty, need to err on the side

v

of extreme caution, even to the point of apparently contradicting the received wisdom in that field.

This being said, some of the contraindications in this book remain controversial, and demonstrate the difficulty of setting guidelines in an area where consensus is hard to achieve. The seesaw of opinion regarding the appropriate use of certain herbs is often impelled by an unquestioning overreliance on research outcomes to the detriment of clinical practice and traditional use. For example, the supposed properties of all preparations of a particular plant may be extrapolated from research on individual plant constituents or specific plant extracts. The resulting distortions reflect both a lack of scientific rigor and a casual disregard of tradition.

Echinacea is a case in point. The host of myths now circulating about this herb—that it is a T-cell activator, or leads to increased TNF-$\alpha$ and is thus contraindicated in AIDS—are based on *in vitro* research on Echinacea polysaccharides, which are not present in alcoholic extracts. Even where the polysaccharides are present in small quantities—as in the expressed juice—they are largely destroyed in the colon by bacterial activity. Research shows that polysaccharide absorption through the gut is about 1%.

For these reasons—and because clinical practice shows, for instance, that Echinacea often benefits patients with autoimmune disease—the contraindications given for Echinacea must be regarded as highly contentious, as Dr. Brinker indicates. The same goes for chaparral and other 'controversial' herbs on which the jury is still out. If these caveats are borne in mind, this book will prove a valuable resource, not only for those unversed in botanical medicine, but also for phytotherapists, whose patients frequently take herbal remedies in combination with prescription drugs.

Colin Nicholls
Editor, British Journal of Phytotherapy
Tunbridge Wells, July 1997

# Introduction

The increasing popularity and use of herbs as flavorful beverages, dietary supplements, and botanical medicines has led to a variety of concerns by health care practitioners, regulating agencies and the public. More frequently these days, herbal preparations are utilized in conjunction with limitations in a person's health. Sometimes they are used in addition to conventional pharmaceutical medicines.

In cases which are not being monitored by a knowledgeable prescriber, herbal use can lead to the inappropriate application of a supplement or remedy in individuals with conditions which may be aggravated by the effect of the herbal product. Another possibility is that the herb or herbs may interfere with medications a person may be using. An herb-aggravated condition or herb/drug interference may not even be associated with the original reason for taking the herbs. A person may consider the connection between their herb use and other medical problems as coincidental, if they appreciate the connection at all. Even for the trained and knowledgeable prescriber organized information associating herbs with undesirable applications has not been readily available.

Appropriate advise is essential to prevent the avoidable harm that may result from inadvertent misapplication of medicinally-active herb products. The need for knowledgeable recommendations exists beyond the current major providers of herbal products and therapies such as herbalists and health food store proprietors. As the herbal market expands more into pharmacies, pharmacists familiar with the patient's medications especially need to be informed about possible risks associated with herbal use.

Pharmacists act as the conventional gate-keepers of medical self-help not only by providing prescription and over-the-counter medicines to patients but also by supplying information on their appropriate use. They are the most accessible personnel knowledgeable in medicines. This knowledge needs to be expanded to include herbs as both potentially beneficial and as disruptive agents.

Physicians also need to be familiar with herbs used by their patients, whether they prescribe them or not. In 1993 fully one third of patients reported utilizing unconventional medical therapy annually, and this number is certain to increase. For doctors who utilize herbal therapeutics in combination with other forms or methods of treatment, this book is even more pertinent. The information on drug interactions may be applied not only to help eliminate therapeutic interference but to aid in reaching a complementary therapeutic balance of activity from both pharmaceutical and botanical agents.

For these reasons a reference book on herbal contraindications and drug interactions is essential at this time for all those whose work in the medical field brings them into contact with individuals who receive or desire herbal therapy to maintain or enhance their health.

This book is also useful to anyone who wants to avoid complicating their current condition or treatment by the self-administration of inappropriate herbs. Terminology that is understandable for the general public is highlighted in bold type. Further technical information to describe the nature of the incompatibilities is provided for health care professionals with numerical superscripts to reference the sources of this information in the medical and scientific literature.

The herbs considered in this book are those which are commonly available without a prescription. The available forms of these products include crude, dried plant parts used to make herbal teas, bottled tablets or encapsulated powders, and commercially-prepared liquid extracts. Only botanical products administered orally, externally, or by inhalation are considered here; injectable items lie outside the scope of this text. Plants whose relative toxicity and/or illegality prevent their being sold to the general public are not considered. The proper use of markedly toxic plants and those requiring a prescription is dependent on the judgment of licensed physicians who can make the assessments necessary to assure their correct application.

Essential (volatile, aromatic) oils concentrated by distillation from otherwise safe plants are also not considered here, since they are so potent as to require special training and considerations for their safe and appropriate use.

Commonly used plants that are generally safe, but have a potential for side effects when taken in excessive doses, are marked with an asterisk (*). To help assure safe use of these plants it is recommended that a companion text on the toxicology of botanical medicines be consulted.

The contraindications listed apply to each herb most accurately when the herb is used alone. When a botanical remedy is taken in conjunction with other herbs or agents that modify or counteract its undesirable effect(s), its use may be rendered safer. This remains a matter of clinical judgment for the knowledgeable prescriber. The contraindications given herein apply to the use of a full therapeutic dose of preparations yielding significant amounts of active constituents. The use of flavorful dried herbs to make mild beverage teas or for culinary purposes may be entirely safe in conditions in which their therapeutic use, requiring a larger dose or a more concentrated form, is contraindicated.

Compared to the amount of crude herb or simple herbal tea, the use of moderately concentrated herbal solid extracts or alcoholic extracts, respectively, requires significantly smaller doses to produce similar effects. For the fluid preparations this is particularly true when considering the effects of volatile oil or resinous components which are much more soluble in alcohol than in water. The powdered and encapsulated crude herbs would be less active in most cases because the absorption of their components tends to be slower and less complete.

ix

An exception to both of the above generalizations would be the drug interactions with crude herbs having hydrocolloidal carbohydrate components (i.e., gums and mucilages) that are soluble in water but relatively insoluble in alcohol. These poorly-absorbed, water-soluble compounds are even more apt to bind to other drugs and interfere with their absorption if taken in their whole or powdered form (e.g., flax seed or marshmallow root) than as liquid extracts.

Plants are listed alphabetically according to the common names by which they are known throughout most of America. This is followed by the corresponding Latin scientific name(s) which identifies the plant more accurately. There follows (in the body of the text) a list of other common names, mostly American and British, that apply to that plant in various locales or settings. Most plants also have common names listed in German and French, many in Spanish, and some in other European or native American languages. In the appendices the plants are listed only by their main American common name and the Latin scientific binomial. Though at this time most herbs are known and sold by one of their common names, identification solely by means of a common name is extremely unreliable since several herbs can share the same designation. The Latin name for each plant is unique and is therefore preferable for correct identification.

Sources of information for this text include not only current scientific laboratory research and pharmacological animal studies but also the discoveries of empirical medicine in this country and abroad from a time when plant remedies were still a major part of conventional practice. This clinically-tested information on herb activities or interactions is based on medical observations of humans. Folk medicine has also helped to identify certain herbal actions that have become a part of established medical knowledge. In this way, for example, it was discovered that the use of certain emmenagogues can have an early abortifacient effect. Such observations taken in conjunction with recent findings identifying uterine stimulant activity help to develop parameters to limit their use appropriately.

The contraindications and drug interactions listed in this text are in reference to the crude herb or its simple extracts unless otherwise noted. For cases in which a particular major constituent is known to produce the effect under consideration, it is duly noted. The descriptions of activities of various chemical constituents is intended to help reveal the rationale behind particular restrictions.

An attempt has been made to be as inclusive as possible in establishing contraindications to the point of being overly cautious. This is particularly true in regard to herbs considered to be contraindicated in pregnancy. However, this is not to imply that each and every medicinal herb with potential contraindications or drug interactions are included in this text or that all possible contraindicated conditions are listed for each herb presented.

A few vitamins and minerals have been listed under "Drug Interactions," since they may be prescribed in deficiency syndromes or in high doses for therapeutic purposes. However, this text does not include contraindications and drug interactions of such nutritional supplements *per se*.

The appendices address potential problematic categories of plants based on their common properties or constituents. The listed plants are discussed in relation to pathological conditions or classes of medications with which they should not ordinarily be used. In some cases they may still be used with care under the supervision of a physician.

The appendices include a number of plants that are not listed in the body of the text. These include plants that are less common, that are prescription items, and/or that have significant toxicity. Precautions may be listed for plants in the appendices that do not appear in the body of the text if the relationship is not as certainly deleterious or the pertinent plant part is not documented.

The index includes all common and scientific names to facilitate locating information on a plant which is known by numerous terms throughout the Western world. The index also lists in bold type the conditions having herbal contraindications and medications that may be interfered with. This allows the information to be accessed by those interested in a particular plant, condition, or type of medication in regard to each individual's personal situation. Though attempting to be as comprehensive as possible in listing incompatibilities for the most commonly used herbs, invariably some items will have been excluded. As the action and interaction of herbs on pathological conditions and other medications continues to be explored and investigated, the breadth and depth of knowledge will continue to develop. Even if the current information is incomplete, this is not a sufficient reason to neglect presenting it. Hopefully, it will at least help to identify the limitations in our understanding so that these can be more adequately addressed.

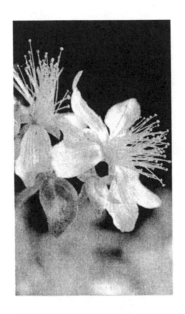

# CONTRAINDICATIONS
# &
# DRUG INTERACTIONS

Designation of
Contraindications, Drug Interactions
and Potential Side Effects

Herbs—Contraindications
and Drug Interactions

# Designation of "Contraindications," "Drug Interactions" and Potential Side Effects

**Contraindication** typically describes an absolute limitation on the use of a particular medicinal substance. It identifies a medical application as improper or undesirable in a particular context. For medicinal herbs, many of which are also used as culinary flavorings for food or as recreational beverage teas, contraindication is often a relative restriction based upon the size of the dose and/or the extent of its use.

Moderate or occasional consumption of herbs may be safe in "contraindicated" conditions that, if taken in large medicinal doses and/or on a continual basis, could possibly result in disagreeable effects. The listing of any potentially dangerous application as a contraindication in this book is a conscious attempt to avoid all foreseeable problems by erring, if misjudgments are made, on the side of safety. "First, do no harm."

Knowledgeable physicians or expert herbal practitioners may decide, in the context of their education and experience, to use particular herbs for individuals with conditions listed here as contraindicated for those herbs. The clinical judgments of such experts for specific patients cannot be condemned solely on the basis of the general statements being made in this text, since the risk of adverse effects can vary based upon timing, dosage, and duration of treatment and auxiliary methods or herbs employed.

Educated and experienced practitioners astute in the art of prescribing may be able to overcome certain contraindications or undesirable drug interactions by making other therapeutic accommodations or adjustments in treatment. The general public, however, should follow all safety guidelines unless they are otherwise directed by an expert in herbal prescribing whose care they are under.

Minute dilutions of plant extracts used as homeopathic medicines do not produce effects equivalent to the undiluted extracts (mother tinctures) or to the plants themselves. Therefore, homeopathic dilutions do not necessarily share the contraindications for those plants.

**Drug interaction** typically refers to a detrimental effect due to the combining of one therapeutic agent with another. However, not all interactions of herbs with drugs are problematic. In this text, therefore, documented examples are included where using an herbal substance with certain pharmaceuticals can enhance the efficacy and/or reduce the toxicity of the drug(s).

**Side effects** are a concern when certain herbs are taken in excessive doses. An **asterisk (\*)** in front of a herb's scientific name denotes that the herb has a possible toxicity.

Consideration of potential side effects and toxic doses requires a separate treatment of these issues. This type of information is available in sources such as *The Toxicology of Botanical Medicines*, Revised 2nd Edition (See reference 2).

# Herbs—
# Contraindications and
# Drug Interactions

## ACACIA

*Acacia senegal* gummy exudate
(gum arabic, Cape gum, Egyptian thorn, gum mimosa, gummi arabicum)

### Drug Interactions

1) gelatinized by solutions of ferric (not ferrous) salts of **iron**[9]

2) insoluble in **alcohol** of greater than 50% concentration[9]

3) reduces rate of absorption of **oral drugs**[4]

## ALFALFA

*Medicago sativa* plant
(buffalo herb, lucerne, purple medic)

### Contraindications

1) **pregnancy** due to the uterine stimulant action on animal uteri of the constituent stachydrine in variety *Medicago sativa* var. *italica*[74]

### Drug Interactions

1) increase rate of metabolism of **xenobiotics** in the liver by increasing the activity of hepatic microsomal mixed-function oxidase reactions[3]

## ALOES

*Aloe* spp. dried leaf exudate (not the gel or juice) (cape aloe, barbados aloe, curacao aloe, bombay aloe, acibar)

### Contraindications

1) profuse **menstruation** or **bleeding between periods**[1,2] due to increase in blood flow to the uterus[5]

2) **pregnancy**[1,2,4,5,24] due to emmenogogue[2,5,6,74] and abortifacient effects[2,4,74]

3) **nursing mothers**[24] due to its purging effect on the suckling child[4,5,6]

4) **stomach inflammation** or **intestinal inflammation** with irritation and/or congestion[1,2,5,24] or intestinal inflammatory diseases such as **ulcerative colitis** or **Crohn's disease**[6] due to irritating effect of anthranoid derivatives (aloins)[2,6]

5) inflamed **hemorrhoids**[1,2,5,24] due to possible induction of stenosis, thrombosis, and prolapse[6]

6) **children** younger than 12 due to depletion of water and electrolytes[6]

7) **extended use** for more that 8 - 10 days due to loss of peristalsis from intestinal smooth muscle and mesenteric plexi damage[6]

8) **intestinal obstruction** due to stimulation of peristalsis by the anthroquinones[4,6]

9) **kidney disorders**[24] since excessive doses can cause nephritis[2]

### Drug Interactions

1) overuse or misuse can cause potassium loss leading to increased toxicity of **cardiac glycosides**[4,6] such as those in *Adonis, Convallaria, Urginea,*[2,6] *Helleborus, Strophanthus,* and *Digitalis*[2]

2) reduced absorption of **oral drugs** due to a decrease in bowel transit time[6]

3) aggravates potassium loss caused by **diuretics**[6]

## ANGELICA

*Angelica archangelica* plant and root

(European angelica, garden angelica, root of the Holy Ghost, engelwurzel, heiligenwurzel, angelique)

### Contraindications

1) plant during **pregnancy** due to its emmenagogue effect[2,74]

2) root in **peptic ulcer** [6] due to its stimulation of gastric acid secretion[4]

3) plant/root in **ultraviolet light** or **solarium therapy** due to photosensitizing furanocoumarins[4,6]

## ANISE

*Pimpinella anisum* fruit

(aniseed, common anise, anis)

### Contraindications

1) **allergic hypersensitivity** due to potential for occasional reaction[6]

## ARNICA

*\*Arnica montana* flowers

(leopardsbane, wolfsbane, common arnica, mountain arnica, mountain tobacco, arnika)

### Contraindications

1) tincture **full strength externally**[7] on **hypersensitive skin**[2,5,6] or **broken skin**[1,2,5] due to the irritating volatile oils (thymol, thymol

methylether and β-tepineol) contained in the tincture[3]

2) **prolonged use externally** leading to hypersensitivity (allergic dermititis) from the sesqiterpene lactones (helenalin methacrylate, helenalin acetate and arnifolin)[3]

3) **internal use** due to the toxic effects on the heart, liver and kidneys of the sesquiterpene lactones and the hepato-enteric irritation caused by essential oil components[3]

4) **pregnancy** due to its uterine stimulant action[2,74]

## ARTICHOKE

*Cynara scolymus* leaf

(globe artichoke, garden artichoke, artischocke, artichaut)

### Contraindications

1) **allergic hypersensitivity** to artichoke or other Asteracea[6]

2) **bile duct obstruction** due to its cholagogue effect[6]

## ASAFETIDA

*Ferula assa-foetida* root

(devil's dung, food of the gods)

### Contraindications

1) **pregnancy** due to its abortifacient effect[2,74] and the emmenogogue effect of its gum-resin[5]

## ASPARAGUS

*Asparagus officinalis* rhizome

(sparrow grass, spargelkraut, asperge)

### Contraindications

1) **kidney inflammation**[6] due to its diuretic effect and irritation to the urinary tract[5]

## BALM

*Melissa officinalis* leaves and flowers

(lemon balm, balm mint, bee balm, blue balm, garden balm, sweet balm, cure-all, dropsy plant, melisse)

### Contraindications

1) **pregnancy** due to its emmenagogue effect[2,3,7,74] as well as its antithyrotropic and antigonadotropic activity[3]

2) **low thyroid** activity due to its antithyrotropic effects[3]

### Drug Interactions

1) increases hypnotic effect of **pentobarbital**[58] and **hexobarbital** due to the sedative activity of the volatile oil[59]

## BALSAM OF TOLU

*Myroxylon balsamum* bark exudate

(tolu balsam, balsam tree, tolubalsambaum, arbre de baume de tolu)

### Contraindications

1) **inflammation** or **feverish conditions**[1] of an active, acute nature due to its stimulant effect on the mucus membranes[5]

## BARBERRY

*Berberis vulgaris* root bark
(European barberry, jaundice berry, pepperidge,
pepperidge bush, sowberry, berberitzenbeeren,
epine vinette, berbero)

### Contraindications

1) **pregnancy** due to the uterine stimulant action
on animal uteri from its alkaloids (berberine,
palmatine, jatorrhizine, columbamine)[2,74]

## BASIL

*Ocymum basilicum* plant
(common basil, sweet basil, St. Josephwort,
basilikum, kleine burgmunze, basilic, albahaca,
bassilico, vol mynte)

### Contraindications

1) **pregnancy**[2,6] due to its emmenagogue[2,74] and
abortifacient effects[74] and the mutagenic action of
its essential oil component (estragole)[6]
2) **nursing mothers** due to the mutagenic effect of
its voltile component estragole[6]
3) for **prolonged use** due to the potentially
carcinogenic effect of estragole[6]

## BAYBERRY

*Myrica cerifera* bark
(wax myrtle, candleberry, tallow shrub, vegetable
tallow, waxberry)

### Contraindications

1) during severe **inflammation**[1] of an acute nature
on mucosa such as in the gastrointestinal tract due
to its local stimulant properties[5]

## BEARBERRY

*Arctostaphylos uva-ursi* leaves

(uva ursi, kinnikinnick, bear's grape, arberry, mealberry, mountain box, mountain cranberry, red bearberry, sagsckhomi, sandberry, upland cranberry, barentraube, bousserole, raisin d'ours, gayuba)

### Contraindications

1) **pregnancy**[2] due to its oxytocic action[2,24]

2) **prolonged use in children** due to possible liver impairment[24]

3) **kidney disorders**[24] possibly due to the urinary excretion of its tannin metabolites[5]

### Drug Interactions

1) **urinary acidifiers** inhibit conversion of arbutin to active hydroquinone, rendering bearberry less effective[4,6]

## BETEL NUT

*\*Areca catechu* seed

(areca nut, betelnutpalme, arequier)

### Contraindications

1) **pregnancy** due to it teratogenic and fetotoxic effects as shown in mice[2,73]

## BIRCH

*Betula pendula* = *Betula alba* leaves

(European birch, white birch, canoe birch, paper birch, hange-birke, birke, bouleau blanc, bouleau ecorce, corteza de abedul , birk, beresa)

### Contraindications

1) **edema** from **heart failure** or **kidney insufficiency** due to inadequate diuretic effect[6]

## BITTER MELON

*Momordica charantia* fruit
(karela, cundeamor, bitter gourd)

### Contraindications

1) **pregnancy** due to the emmenogogue and abortifacient effects of its juice[74]

### Drug Interactions

1) **insulin** dosage may need adjusting due to hypoglycemic effect in diabetic patients[34,35]

## BITTER ORANGE

*Citrus aurantium* ssp. *amara* peel
(Seville orange, sour orange, pomeranzenbaum, bigaradier, oranger amer)

### Contraindications

1) **stomach ulcers** or **intestinal ulcers**[6] due to its tonic effect on the GI tract[5]

## BLACK COHOSH

*\*Cimicifuga racemosa* roots/rhizome
(macrotys, black snakeroot, bugbane, bugwort, rattleroot rattlewort, rattleweed, richweed, squawroot, Amerikanisches wanzenkraut, schwarze schlangenwurzel, actee a grappes, herbe au punaise)

### Contraindications

1) **pregnancy** during the first trimester[2] due to its emmenagogue effect[2,5,7,74]

## BLACK PEPPER

*Piper nigrum* fruit

(pepper)

**Contraindications**

1) **pregnancy** due to its abortifacient effect[2,74]

## BLACK POPLAR

*Populus nigra* buds

(schwarzpappel, peuplier noir)

**Contraindications**

1) **externally in allergic hypersensitivity** to poplar, propolis, Peruvian balsam, or salicylates due to occasional skin reactions[6]

## BLACK RADISH

*Raphanus sativus* var. *niger* root

(schwarzer rettich, radis noir)

**Contraindications**

1) **bile stones**[6] due to its cholagogue effect[7]

## BLADDERWRACK

*Fucus vesiculosus* plant

(seawrack, common seawrack, cut weed, sea kelp, kelpware, black tang, tang, varech vesiculeux)

**Contraindications**

1) **excess thyroid** activity due to high iodine content[4,6]

2) **partial thyroid removal** or **Hashimoto's thyroiditis** due to inducing myxedema by increasing interthyroidal concentrations of iodide which blocks thyroxin formation[39]

## BLAZING STAR
*Aletris farinosa* root
(star grass, ague grass, bitter grass, colic root,
mealy starwort, star root)

### Contraindications
1) **pregnancy** when using large amounts due to its
uterine stimulant action on animal uteri[2,74]

## BLESSED THISTLE
*Cnicus benedictus* plant
(St. Benedict thistle, holy thistle, spotted thistle,
cardin, kardo-benediktenkraut, chardon bevit,
cardo santo)

### Contraindications
1) **allergic hypersensitivity** to this plant or other
Asteracea[6]

## BLOODROOT
*Sanguinaria canadensis* rhizome
(Indian paint, Indian plant, Indian red paint,
pauson, red paint root, red puccoon, red root,
tetterwort, kanadische blutwurzel, sanguinaire)

### Contraindications
1) **pregnancy** due to its emmenogogue effect[7] and
the uterine stimulant action on animal uteri by its
alkaloids (berberine, protopine, chelerythrine)[2,74]

## BLUE COHOSH
*Caulophyllum thalictroides* root
(beechdrops, blueberry, blue ginseng, papoose
root, squaw root, yellow ginseng)

## Contraindications

1) **pregnancy** prior to the ninth month due to its emmenagogue[3,7,10] and abortifacient effects[2,3,6,10,74] and its uterine stimulant activity on animal uteri from its saponin (caulosaponin)[2,3,6,74]

## BOLDO

*Peumus boldus* leaves
(boldu)

## Contraindications

1) **bile duct obstruction** or **serious liver disorders** due to its choleretic activity[4,6] (use with gallstones only after consultation with doctor)[4]

## BONESET

*Eupatorium perfoliatum* plant
(agueweed, crosswort, feverwort, Indian sage, sweating plant, teasel, thoroughwort, vegetable antimony, wood boneset, durchwachsener wasserhanf, herbe a la fievre)

## Contraindications

1) **allergic hypersensitivity** can result in contact dermatitis due to the sesquiterpene lactone constituents that are found in this and other members of the *Eupatorium* genus[10]

## BORAGE

*\*Borago officinalis* plant
(burrage, bugloss, common bugloss, boretsch, bourrache, borraggine, borrana, boraga)

### Contraindications

1) **excessive use** or **prolonged use** due to presence of pyrrolizidine alkaloids that known hepatotoxins and potential carcinogens[6]

(Borage seed oil is safe and does not contain pyrrolizidine alkaloids.)

## BUCHU

*Barosma betulina* leaves

(bookoo, bucco, bucku, short buchu)

### Contraindications

1) **acute genito-urinary tract inflammation**[1,2] due to the glycoside diosmin and essential oil components (diosphenol and pulegone) that can cause mucosal irritation[2,4]

2) **pregnancy**[24] probably due to the high content of the mucosal irritant and uterine stimulant volatile component pulegone[2] found in the spurious *Barosma crenulata* (called oval buchu) that is often used as a substitute[70,71]

## BUCKTHORN

*Rhamnus cathartica* fruit

(common buckthorn, purging buckthorn, waythorn, kreuzdorn, purgierdorn, nerprun, espino cerval)

### Contraindications

1) **intestinal obstruction** due to increased peristalsis from the anthroquinones[4,6]

2) **pregnancy**[4] since high doses of anthroquinones can may stimulate endometrial activity and cause abortion[6]

3) **nursing mothers**[4] since anthroquinones are partly excreted in the milk[6]

4) **intestinal inflammatory diseases** due to the irritation to the mucosa[6]
5) **children** under age 12 due to loss of water and electrolytes[6]
6) **extended use** for more than 8-10 days due to loss of water and electrolytes[6]
7) **abdominal pain** of unknown origin[6] due to possible rupture from contraction of inflamed viscus such as the appendix

### Drug Interactions

1) overuse or misuse can cause potassium loss leading to increased toxicity of **cardiac glycosides**[4,6] such as those in *Adonis, Convallaria, Urginea*[2,6] *Helleborus, Strophanthus,* and *Digitalis*[2]
2) potassium loss may result in hypokalemia when taking **diuretics**[6]
3) reduced absorption of **oral drugs** due to a decrease in bowel transit time[6]

## BUGLEWEED

*Lycopus virginicus, Lycopus europaeus* leaves (sweet bugle, water bugle, water hoarhound, gypsy weed, Paul's betony, green ashangee, archangle, wolf's foot, wolfstrapp, lycope, patte de loup)

### Contraindications

1) **low thyroid** activity or **nontoxic goiter** due to its antithyrotropic effects[3,6]
2) **pregnancy** due to its antigonadotropic and antithyrotropic activity[6]
3) **nursing mothers** due to its antiprolactin activity[6]

**Drug Interactions**

1) can interfere with **thyroid hormones**[6] since it blocks conversion of thyroxin to $T_3$ in the liver and interfers with iodine metabolism in the thyroid by inhibiting thyroid stimulating hormone[3]

2) interferes with radioactive **iodine** uptake[6]

## BURDOCK

*Arctium lappa* root

(bardana, burr seed, clotbur, cocklebur, grass burdock, hardock, hareburr, hurrburr, turkey burrseed, kletterwurzel, grote klette, bardane, sampazo)

**Contraindications**

1) **pregnancy** due to its oxytocic effect[10] and uterine stimulant action on animal uteri[2,74]

## BUTTERBUR

*\*Petasites hybridus = Petasites officinalis* rhizome (butterfly dock, grobblattriger huflattich, rote pestwurz, petasite)

**Contraindications**

1) **pregnancy** due to its emmenogogue effect[74] and its content of hepatotoxic/genotoxic/ carcinogenic pyrrolizidine alkaloids[6]

2) **nursing mothers** due to its content of toxic pyrrolizidine alkaloids[6]

## BUTTERCUP

*Ranunculus* spp. plant
(crowfoot, gold cup)

### Contraindications

1) **pregnancy** due to the uterine stimulant action
on animal uteri by its component seratonin[2,74]

## CALAMUS

*Acorus calamus* root
(sweet flag, grass myrtle, myrtle flag, sweet grass,
sweet myrtle, sweet rush, kalmus, acore vrai,
calamo aromatico, acoro aromatico)

### Contraindications

1) **pregnancy**[2] due to its emmenagogue effect[2,7,74]

## CALENDULA

*Calendula officinalis* flowers
(garden marigold, holigold, marigold, Mary bud,
goldbloom, pot marigold, ringelblume, souci des
champs, fleurs de tous les mois, mejorana,
claveton, flaminquillo, fior d'ogni)

### Contraindications

1) **pregnancy** due to its emmenagogue[2,3,74] and
abortifacient effects[2]

### Drug Interactions

1) sedative effect[55] increases **hexobarbital**
sleeping time due to the saponoside components[56]

## CALIFORNIA POPPY

*Eschscholtzia californica* plant
(yellow poppy, goldpoppy, copa de oro, amapola
amarilla, amapola de California, cululuk,
Kalifornischer goldmohn)

### Contraindications

1) **pregnancy** due to uterine stimulant effect shown by alkaloid constituent (cryptopine) on animal uteri[6]

### Drug Interactions

1) enhanced the hypnotic effect induced by **pentobarbital**[66,67]

## CAMPHOR TREE

*Cinnamomum camphora* bark

(laurel camphor, camphor laurel, kampferbaum, camphrier)

### Contraindications

1) **pregnancy** due to its emmenagogue effect[2,74] and the uterine stimulant activity[74] and fetocidal effects when isolated camphor is used[2]

2) on **damaged skin**[6] due to the rubefacient effect of its monoterpene camphor[2]

3) use of camphor near the **nose of infants** or small **children**[6] since its inhalation and absorption in small doses can result in CNS overstimulation and seizures[2]

## CASCARA SAGRADA

*Rhamnus purshiana* aged bark

(California buckthorn, sacred bark, chittim bark, Amerikanischer faulbaum)

### Contraindications

1) chronic **intestinal inflammatory diseases** or **intestinal ulcers**[2,6,24] due to the irritation and inflammation of the bowel caused by the anthroquinone glycosides (cascarosides)[2,6]

2) **nursing mothers** due to the excretion of anthroquinones in breast milk[3,4,6]

3) **menstruation**[3] due to possible stimulation of endometrial activity[6]

4) acute **diarrhea** due to the increase hydration of the stools caused by cascarosides[3]

5) generally **debilitated subjects**[3] due to loss of water and electrolytes[6]

6) **intestinal obstruction** due to stimulation of peristalsis by the anthroquinones[3,4,6]

7) **abdominal pain** of unknown origin[3,6] due to possible rupture from contraction of inflamed viscus such as the appendix

8) **children** under 12 years of age due to loss of water and electrolytes[6]

9) **extended use** for more than 8-10 days due to possible damage to intestinal muscle and mesenteric plexi[6]

10) **pregnancy**[4,24] due to stimulation of the endometrium which may provoke abortion[6]

11) **recent bark** aged less than 1 year due to its anthrone content leading to gastrointestinal upset[6,7]

## Drug Interactions

1) overuse or misuse can cause potassium loss leading to increased toxicity of **cardiac glycosides**[4,6] such as those in *Adonis, Convallaria, Urginea,*[2,6] *Helleborus, Strophanthus,* and *Digitalis*[2]

2) reduced absorption of **oral drugs** due to a decrease in bowel transit time[6]

3) aggravates potassium loss caused by **diuretics**[6]

## CASSIA CINNAMON

*Cinnamomum aromaticum = Cinnamomum cassia* bark

(cassia, cassia bark, Chinesischer zimtbaum, cannellier de Chine)

### Contraindications

1) **pregnancy**[2,6] due to its emmenagogue and abortifacient effects[2,74]

2) **allergic hypersensitivity** to cinnamon or Peruvian balsam[6]

### Drug Interactions

1) reduced absorption of **tetracycline** taken with the powdered bark occurs due to adsorption by the bark powder[45]

## CASTOR BEAN

*Ricinus communis* oil

(Mexico seed, oil plant, palma Christi, castor-oil plant, wunderbaum, bofareira)

### Contraindications

1) **intestinal obstruction** or unexplained **stomach ache** due to its gastric irritant[4] and purgative effects[5,7]

2) **prolonged use** due to potential for serious electolyte loss[6]

### Drug Interactions

1) electrolyte loss from frequent use may potentiate **cardiac glycosides**[6] such as those in *Adonis, Convallaria, Urginea,*[2,6] *Helleborus, Strophanthus,* and *Digitalis*[2]

## CATNIP

*Nepeta cataria* leaves and flowers
(catmint, catnep, catrup, catswort, field balm,
echtes katzenkraut, katzenminze, cataire)

### Contraindications

1) **pregnancy** due to its emmenagogue and
abortifacient effects[2,74]

## CAYENNE

*\*Capsicum frutescens* fruit
(Africa pepper, bird pepper, chili pepper, cockspur
pepper, goat's pepper, pod pepper, red pepper,
Spanish pepper, Zanzibar pepper, cayennepfeffer,
piment de cayenne)

### Contraindications

1) **asthma**, when consumed acutely by itself or
when extract containing capsaicin is inhaled, due
to the immediate bronchoconstriction[3]
2) **externally over damaged skin** due to irritant
properties[6]
3) **externally on hypersensitive skin** due to
possible (though rare) allergic reactions[6]
4) **stomach ulcers** or **stomach inflammation**[3,24]
because its component capsaicin increases gastric
acid production and can cause mucosal exfoliation
and hemorrhage[3]
5) chronic **bowel irritation**[24] due to the mucosal
irritant and stimulant properties of capsaicin[3]

## CEDARWOOD

*Juniperus virginiana, Juniperus ashei* heartwood
(Virginia cedarwood, eastern red cedar, red
juniper, Texas cedarwood, Ashe juniper)

**Drug Interactions**

1) inhalation of fragrance containing cedrol or cedrene reduces effects of **hexobarbital** and **dicoumarol** due to induction of microsomal enzymes including aniline hydroxylase, sulfanilamide acetylase, neoprontosil azoreductase, heptachlor epoxidase and zoxazolamine hydroxylase[6]

## CELANDINE

*Chelidonium majus* root and plant
(great celandine, garden celandine, tetterwort, greater celandine, schollkraut, chelidoine)

**Contraindications**

1) **pregnancy** due to its uterine stimulant activity[3] and content of alkaloids (chelidonine, sparteine, protopine, chelerythrine and berberine) that act as uterine stimulants in animal uteri[2,3,74]

## CELERY

*Apium graveolens* seeds
(garden celery, kuchen-sellerie, sellerie, ache des marais, celeri)

**Contraindications**

1) acute **kidney inflammation**[1,4,24] due to irritation caused by excretion of its volatiles oil components (monoterpenes and phthalides) in urine[3,4]

2) **pregnancy**[2,3,7,24] due to the emmenogogue[7] and abortifacient effects and uterine stimulant activity on animal uteri by the seeds and their volatile oil[2,3,74]

3) **ultraviolet light** or **solarium therapy** due to phototoxic furanocoumarins[4,6]

## CHAMOMILE, GERMAN

*Matricaria recutita = Matricaria chamomilla* plant (wild chamomile, camomile, Hungarian chamomile, pin heads, kamillen, echte kamille, kleine kamille, feldkamille, fleur de camomile, camomille, matricaire, camomilla, manzanilla)

### Contraindications

1) **pregnancy** due to its emmenagogue effect[2,74] [The flowers, the part most commonly used, are safe except for a few rare cases of allergic skin reactions.][4,6,64]

## CHAMOMILE, ROMAN

*Chamaemelum nobile = Anthemis nobilis* plant (garden chamomile, English chamomile, sweet chamomile, camomile, ground apple, low chamomile, whig plant, Romischc kamille, grote kamille, fleur de camomille romaine manzanilla)

### Contraindications

1) **pregnancy** due to its emmenogogue and abortifacient effects and that of its volatile oil[2,74] [The flowers, the part most commonly used, are safe except for mild allergic skin reactions.][64]

## CHAPARRAL

*Larrea tridentata, Larrea divaricata* leaves (creosote bush, greasewood, gobernadora, hediondilla, tasajo, jarillo, shoegoi, ya-temp, geroop, kovanau)

### Contraindications

1) history of **liver damage**[16] due to its possible hepatotoxic effect[3,6,16]

2) **allergic hypersensitivity** to the plant or its resin[85,86]

## CHASTE TREE

*Vitex agnus-castus* berries

(hemp tree, keuschbaum, agneau chaste, gatillier)

### Contraindications

1) **pregnancy** due to its emmenagogue effect[3,74]

## CHICORY

*Cichorium intybus* root

(wild chicory, succory, wild succory, wegwarte, cichorie, chicoree, achicoria amarga, cicoria, zikorifa, suikerey)

### Contraindications

1) **pregnancy** due to its emmenagogue and abortifacient effects[2,74]

2) **allergic hypersensitivity** to chicory and other Asteraceae[6]

## CINCHONA

*\*Cinchona* spp. bark

(Peruvian bark, Jesuits' bark, fieberrinde, Chinarinde, quina, quinquina)

### Contraindications

1) **pregnancy**[1,2,6,7] due to its uterine stimulant activity[7,74] and abortifacient effect[2,74] and the oxytocic effects of its alkaloids quinine and quinidine[2,10,74] and its teratogenic (causes visual and auditory defects) activity[2] and the fetotoxic and fetocidal effects of its alkaloids[10]

2) in **cinchonism**[5] where preexisting toxicity
symptoms are present[2] from overdosing or
**prolonged use**[2,6]
3) **allergic hypersensitivity**[6] since one third of
patients are reactive to it[2]
4) acute **inflammation** with **feverish conditions**
or **plethora** (flushed, congested face)[5]
5) **nervous irritation, vascular irritation,**  or
active **hemorrhage**[5]
6) **nursing mothers** since its alkaoids (quinine,
quinidine) are excreted in breast milk[2]
7) **stomach ulcers** or **intestinal ulcers**[6] or **amebic
dysentery**[1] due to its grastrointestinal irritant
effect[5]

### Drug Interactions
1) potentiation of **coumarin derivatives**[6]

## CINNAMON

*Cinnamomum verum = Cinnamomum zeylanicum*
bark
(Ceylon cinnamon, zimt, cannelle)

### Contraindications
1) **pregnancy**[2,4,6] due to the emmenagogue effect[2]
of its volatile oil[74]
2) **allergic hypersensitivity** to cinnamon[4,6] due to
its phellandrene content[10] or to Peru balsam[4,6]
probably due to its cinnamein content[10]
3) **stomach ulcers** or **intestinal ulcers**[6] due to its
stomachic effect[5]

## COCOA

*Theobroma cacao* seed

(cacao, chocolate tree)

### Contraindications

1) **allergic hypersensitivity** may result in migraine and/or skin reactions[6]

2) **heart disorders** due to cardiac effects of theobromine and caffeine[10]

### Drug Interactions

1) excessive amounts of chocolate taken with **monoamine oxidase inhibitors** can cause a hypertensive crisis

## COFFEE

*\*Caffea arabica* beans

(mocha, java, cafe, espresso)

### Contraindications

1) acute **kidney inflammation**[1,8] since the diuretic effect of caffeine increase the urinary output[2,5,8]

2) high-grade **inflammation**[1] possibly due to caffeine's CNS stimulant effects causing restlessness and insomnia[2,8]

3) **pregnancy** when taken in large amounts since caffeine (in doses of more than 600 mg) can have abortifacient[2] and teratogenic effects[2,8,10]

4) excess **stomach acid**[2] or **duodenal ulcers** due to increased gastric acid secretion from caffeine[8]

5) **heart disorders** due to acute and/or excessive caffeine consumption increasing heart rate and causing arrhythmias[8,10]

6) **psychological disorders** since caffeine can aggravate depression or induce anxiety neurosis[8]

**Drug Interactions**
1) possible reduced absorption of **oral drugs** taken simultaneously[6]
2) **iron** absorption is inhibited[8]
3) **contraceptives** and **cimetidine** increase the effect of caffeine[8]
4) increased thermogenesis and weight loss due to a reduction of body fat when caffeine is combined with **ephedrine**[18,19] as well as agitation, tremors, and insomnia[19]
5) excessive caffeine taken with **monoamine oxidase inhibitors** can cause a hypertensive crisis

## COLA

*Cola nitida* seed
(kola, kolatier)

**Contraindications**
1) **stomach ulcers** or **duodenal ulcers**[6] due to gastric stimulant effect of caffeine[2,8]
2) **heart disorders** due to acute and/or excessive caffeine consumption increasing heart rate and causing arrhythmias[8,10]

**Drug Interactions**
1) effect enhanced by **psychoanaleptic drugs** and other **caffeine**-containing beverages[6]
2) **contraceptives** and **cimetidine** increase the effect of caffeine[8]
3) increased thermogenesis and weight loss due to a reduction of body fat when caffeine is combined with sources of **ephedrine**[18,19] as well as agitation, tremors, and insomnia[19]
4) excessive amounts of caffeine taken with **monoamine oxidase inhibitors** can cause a hypertensive crisis

## COLTSFOOT

*Tussilago farfara* leaves
(British tobacco, bullsfoot, coughwort, flower
velure, foal's-foot, horsefoot, horsehoof,
huflattich, brandlattich, pferdefut, pas d'ane,
tussilage, una de caballo)

### Contraindications

1) **pregnancy**[2,4,6] due to its abortifacient effect[2,74]
and content of hepatotoxic pyrrolizidine
alkaloids[4,6]
2) **nursing mothers** due to its content of
hepatotoxic pyrrolizidine alkaloids[4,6]
3) **prolonged use** longer than six weeks per year
due to content of hepatotoxic alkaloids[4]

## COMFREY

*Symphytum officinale* root/leaves
(knitbone, knitback, blackwort, bruisewort, gum
plant, healing herb, salsify, slippery root, wallwort,
beinwell, consoude, wallwurz, beindweld, grand
consoude, oreille d'ane, consuelda mayor,
consolida maggiore, simfit, zinzinnici, sinfit)

### Contraindications

1) **internal use** due to hepatotoxic effects and
carcinogenic activity of it pyrrolizidine alkaloids[3,4]
2) on **broken skin**[4,6] to avoid excessive
percutaneous absorption of toxic pyrrolizidine
alkaloids which is typically low on intact skin[37]
3) **pregnancy** due to fetal hepatotoxicity resulting
from transferral from mother of toxic pyrrolizidine
alkaloids[38]

4) **nursing mothers** due to infant hepatotoxicity resulting from transferral from mother of toxic pyrrolizidine alkaloids[38]

## COTTON

*Gossypium herbaceum* fresh root bark

**Contraindications**
1) **pregnancy**[2] due to its oxytocic,[10] emmenogogue, and abortifacient effects[2,5,6,7,74,75]

## CRUCIFER

*Brassica* spp. heads or leaves
(broccoli; cabbage; kale; collards; mustard; turnip)

**Drug Interactions**
1) **warfarin** is rendered ineffective by regular consumption of broccoli or green, leafy vegetables that are high in vitamin K[32,33]

## CUBEB

*\*Piper cubeba* unripe fruit
(Java pepper, tailed cubebs, tailed pepper)

**Contraindications**
1) acute **inflammation**[1,5] of mucosal surfaces, especially **urinary tract inflammation**,[5] due to the local irritating effect of its volatile hydrocarbon (cadinene)[2,5,6]

## DANDELION

*Taraxacum officinale* = *Taraxacum dens-leonis* root
(blowball, cankerwort, lion's tooth, prient's crown, puffball, swine snout, white endive, wild endive, lowenzahn, dent de lion, pissenlit, diente de leon)

## Contraindications

1) acute **stomach inflammation** or **bowel irritation**[1,5] due to its stomachic effect of stimulating gastric hyperacidity[4,5]

2) **digestive weakness**[1,5] because of resulting dyspepsia, flatulence, pain, and diarrhea[5] possibly due to its choleretic and cholagogue effects on the liver and gall bladder[3]

3) **bile duct obstruction** or **biliary inflammation**[4,6,24] due to the cholagogue effect[4,6]

4) **gallstones**[4] due to its cholagogue effect[4,6]

5) **gall bladder inflammation** with pus[4,6,24] due to its cholagogue effect[4,6]

6) **intestinal obstruction**[4,6,24] due to its gastrointestinal stimulation[5]

7) **allergic hypersensitivity** to other Asteraceae such as chamomile, yarrow, and/or arnica[6]

# DEVIL'S CLAW

*Harpagophytum procumbens* root
(grapple plant, teufelskralle, trampelklette, griffe du diable)

## Contraindications

1) **stomach inflammation,**[24] **stomach ulcers,**[4,6,24] and **duodenal ulcers**[4,6] due to its bitter iridoid substances (harpagoside, procumbide) stimulating stomach acid secretion[4]

2) **gallstones** due to its choleretic effect[4]

# DILL

*Anethum graveolens* fruit
(dilly, garden dill, aneth)

## Contraindications

1) **pregnancy** due to its emmenagogue effect[74]

## DYERS WEED

*Genista tinctoria* plant
(dyer's broom, dyer's greenweed, dyer's whin,
furze, green broom, greenweed, waxen woad,
woad waxen, wood waxen, farberginster, genet de
teinturies)

### Contraindications

1) **high blood pressure**[4,6,7] due to its
vasoconstrictive activity[7]

## ECHINACEA

*Echinacea* spp. herb juice/root
(purple coneflower, coneflower, combflower,
Sampson root, black Sampson, sonnenhut,
igelkopfwurzel, racine d'echinacea)

### Contraindications

1) "in principle," **progressive conditions** such as
**multiple sclerosis,**[4,6,17] **collagenosis**[4,17] (possibly
due to stimulation of fibroblasts[82]), **leukosis,**[4,17]
and **auto-immune disorders**[4] (probably due to
non-specific stimulation of the immune response[83]),
**AIDS** or **HIV infection**[4] (probably due to
polymeric compounds such as arabinogalactans
(precipitates removed from filtered alcoholic
extracts) inducing secretion by macrophages of
tumor necrosis factor[83] which is elevated in the
serum of patients with AIDS cachexia), and
**tuberculosis**[4,6,17] (probably since arabinogalactan
constituents are similar to those in *Mycobacteria*
cell walls associated with cell-mediated
suppression of lymphocyte responses in
tuberculosis[87])

## ELECAMPANE

*Inula helenium* root
(elfdock, elfwort, horse elder, horseheal, scabwort, echter alant, aunee, ala)

### Contraindications

1) **allergic hypersensitivity** (contact dermatitis) to its sesquiterpene lactone (alantolactone) or similar cross-reactive substances[4]

## EUCALYPTUS

*\*Eucalyptus* spp. leaves
(blue gum, schonmutz, blauer gommibaum, eukalyptus, gommier bleu, eucalytpo, setma ag, kafur ag)

### Contraindications

1) **low blood pressure**[1] due to hypotensive effect in large doses[2]

2) acute desquamative **kidney inflammation**[1,2] due to irritation from urinary excretion of volatile oil (eucalyptol)[2] and diuretic effect of large doses of the volatile oil[5]

3) **stomach inflammation, biliary inflammation,** or **intestinal inflammation** due to irritation of the mucosa by volatile constituents[4,6]

4) serious **liver disorders** due to the hepatic metabolism of volatile constituents[4,6]

5) oral use or inhalation of essential oil by **children** under age 2[6] due to potential toxicity[2]

### Drug Interactions

1) consumption of the leaves or inhalation of essential oil induces hepatic microsomal mixed-function oxidase enzyme induction[6,28,36] which can increase the rate of metabolism and clearance of drugs such as **pentobarbital, aminopyrine,** and

**amphetamine**, thereby reducing the length of time they are effective[28]

2) microsomal mixed-function oxidase induction can increase the toxicity of plants containing **pyrrolizidine alkaloids** such as *Senecio longilobus* and *Senecio jacobaea*[36]

## FENNEL

*Foeniculum vulgare* fruit
(large fennel, sweet fennel, Florence fennel, wild fennel, fenchel, fenouille, aneth fenouil, hinojo)

### Contraindications

1) **pregnancy** due to the emmenagogue effect,[2,4,14,74] especially for concentrated form such as the essential oil,[6] and phytoestrogen activity of its volatile oil components (anethole, dianethole, photanethole)[14]

2) essential oil for infants or small **children**[6] due to its potential toxicity[2]

## FENUGREEK

*Trigonella foenum-graecum* seed
(bird's foot, Greek hayseed, bockshornklee, fenugrec, fenogreco, mayti)

### Contraindications

1) **pregnancy** due to its emmenagogue and abortifacient effects and its uterine stimulant action on animal uteri[2,74]

### Drug Interactions

1) mucilage coats GI mucosa and retards absorption of **oral drugs**[4]

## FEVERFEW

*Tanacetum parthenium = Chrysanthemum parthenium* plant
(featherfew, febrifuge plant, mutterkraut, camomille grande)

### Contraindications

1) **pregnancy** due to its emmenagogue effect[2,3,74]

## FLAX

*Linum usitatissimum* seeds
(linseed, lint bells, winterlien, leinsamen, flachssamen, grain de lin, lino, lino usuale, keten, bazen, tesi-mosina, alashi, sufulsi, hu-ma-esze)

### Contraindications

1) open **wounds** or **abraded surfaces**[1] possibly to prevent adherence and retention of whole seeds in wounds if used as a poultice

2) **intestinal obstruction**[4,6] to avoid dangerous impaction of bowels

3) **pregnancy** due to emmenagoue effect[2,74]

### Drug Interactions

1) possible reduced absorption of **oral drugs**[4,6] due to its mucilage[4]

## FRAGRANT SUMACH

*Rhus aromatica* root bark
(sweet sumach)

### Contraindications

1) **inflammation**[1,5] of such organs as the intestines, kidneys, uterus, and lungs due to irritating effect of its volatiles oil locally and during excretion[5]

## FRANGULA

*Rhamnus frangula* bark
(alder buckthorn, alder dogwood, arrow-wood,
black alder dogwood, black alder tree, black
dogwood, European black alder, European
buckthorn, Persian berries, faulbaumrinde,
gelbholzrinde, zweckenbaumrinde, bourdaine,
ecorce defrangule, ecorce d'aune noir)

### Contraindications

1) **bowel obstruction** due to the stimulation of peristalsis by its anthrone derivatives (glucofrangulins)[4,6]

2) **intestinal inflammatory diseases**[6,24] due to irritation from the anthroquinones[6]

3) **pregnancy**[4,24] due to possible endometrial stimulation resulting in abortion[6]

4) **nursing mothers**[4] due to passage of anthroquinones into breast milk[6]

5) **children** under 12 years of age due to the water and electrolyte loss[6]

6) **extended use** for more than 8-10 days due to damage to the intestinal smooth muscle and mesenteric plexi[6]

7) **recent bark** of less than 1 year due to its anthrone content leading to gastrointestinal upset[6,7]

8) **ulcers**[24] or **abdominal pain** of unknown origin[6] due to possible rupture from contraction of inflamed viscus such as the appendix

### Drug Interactions

1) overuse or misuse can cause potassium loss leading to increased toxicity of **cardiac glycosides**[4,6] such as those in *Adonis, Convallaria, Urginea,*[2,6] *Helleborus, Strophanthus,* and *Digitalis*[2]

2) reduced absorption of **oral drugs** due to a decrease in bowel transit time[6]

3) aggravates potassium loss caused by **diuretics**[6]

## FRINGE TREE

*Chionanthus virginicus* bark
(gray beard tree, old man's beard, poison ash, snowflower, white fringe)

**Contraindications**

1) **bile duct obstruction**[24] or **bile duct impaction** due to its cholagogue activity[1]

## GARLIC

*Allium sativum* bulbs
(clove garlic, knoblauch, ail)

**Contraindications**

1) acute or chronic **stomach inflammation** or marked irritation or inflammation[1] of other surfaces since the concentrated garlic volatile disulfide components can cause gastroenteritis[2]

2) **pregnancy** due to emmenogogue effect in large amounts and its uterine stimulant action in animal uteri[2,74]

3) **low thyroid** function if high levels of purified constituents are used on a regular basis which can cause a reduced iodine uptake by the thyroid[2]

## GENTIAN

*Gentiana lutea* roots
(yellow gentian, bitter root, bitterwort, pale gentian, enzianwurzel, bitterwurz, fieberwurzel, racine de gentiane, gleber enzian, genciana)

## Contraindications

1) **stomach irritability** or **stomach inflammation**[1,2,5] due to its bitter substances (gentiopicroside, amarogentin) increasing acid secretion by stomach[3]

2) **stomach ulcers** or **duodenal ulcers**[4,6] due to stimulation of acid secretion[4]

## GINGER

*Zingiber officinale* rhizome
(black ginger, race ginger, ingwer, gingembre)

## Contraindications

1) **pregnancy** when taken in large amounts due to its abortifacient effect[2,3,74]

2) **gallstones** due to its cholagogue effect[4]

## GINSENG

*Panax ginseng* root
(Chinese ginseng, panax de chine)

## Drug Interactions

1) concurrent use of **phenelzine** has resulted in manic-like symptoms[26,27]

## GOLDENROD

*Solidago virgaurea* plant
(European goldenrod, goldrute, goldwundkraut, solidage, verge d'or)

## Contraindications

1) chronic **kidney disorders** which require a doctor's supervision[4,6]

2) **edema** from **heart failure** or **kidney insufficiency**[4] since its diuretic effect causes mainly water, not salt, to be excreted[6]

## GOLDENSEAL

*Hydrastis canadensis* roots/rhizome
(eye balm, eye root, ground raspberry, Indian
plant, jaundice root, orangeroot, turmeric root,
yellow puccoon, yellowroot, goldsiegel,
kanadische gelbwurzel)

### Contraindications

1) **pregnancy**[1,2,3,24] due to uterine stimulant action
of its alkaloids (berberine, hydrastine, canadine,
hydrastinine) in certain animal uteri[2,3,74]
2) locally for purulent **ear discharge**[1] due to the
possibility of a ruptured ear drum

## GOTU KOLA

*Centella asiatica* = *Hydrocotyle asiatica* plant
(water pennywort, thick-leaved pennywort, Indian
pennywort, Bevilacqua, asiatischer wassernabel)

### Contraindications

1) **pregnancy** due to its emmenogogue[74] and
abortifacient effects[2,74]

## GUAR GUM

*Cyamopsis* spp. seeds
(guaran)

### Drug Interactions

1) **insulin** requirements for diabetics is reduced
since the gum delays glucose absorption[41]
2) oral absorption of drugs such as **paracetamol,**[42]
**nitrofurantoin,**[43] and **digoxin** is slowed and for
**penicillin** is reduced[44] due to slower gastric
emptying[42] and the viscosity of the gum[43]

## HAWTHORN

*Crataegus* spp. leaves/flowers/fruit
(May tree, quickset, thorn-apple tree, whitethorn,
weitdorn, aubepine, epine blanche)

### Drug Interactions
1) increases activity of cardiotonic plants such as
**digitalis** and **cardiac glycosides including
digitoxin, digoxin** and **g-strophanthin** due to its
polymeric procyanidins while reducing the toxicity
of these glycosides by its coronary vasodilating
and anti-arrhythmic effects[3]

## HEMP AGRIMONY

*\*Eupatorium cannabinum* plant
(waterhemp, throughwort, sweet mandlin, water
mandlin, water maudlin, sweet-smelling trefoil,
Dutch agrimony, Dutch eupatorium, gemeiner
wasserdost, wasserhanf, chanvrin, eupatoire
commune)

### Contraindications
1) **pregnancy** due to its emmenogogue and
abortifacient effects[74] and its content of
hepatotoxic pyrrolizidine alkaloids[6]
2) **nursing mothers** due to its content of toxic
pyrrolizidine alkaloids[6]

## HIBISCUS

*Hibiscus rosa-sinensis* flowers
(rose of China, Chinese hibiscus)

### Contraindications
1) **pregnancy** due to its emmenogogue and
abortifacient effects[2,74]

## HOPS

*Humulus lupulus* strobiles
(hopfen, hopfenzapfen, hopfendrusen, lupulin, houblon)

### Drug Interactions

1) sedative activity increases the sleeping time induced by **pentobarbital**[57]

## HOREHOUND

*Marrubium vulgare* plant
(hoarhound, white horehound, andorn, marrube blanc)

### Contraindications

1) **pregnancy** due to the emmenagogue and abortifacient effects and uterine stimulant action on animal uteri[2,74]

## HORSE CHESTNUT

*Aesculus hippocastanum* seeds
(buckeye, Spanish chestnut, rotkastanie, marronier d'inde)

### Contraindications

1) **bleeding disorders**[24] due to antithrombin activity of its hydroxycoumarin component (aesculin), leading to increased bleeding time[2]

### Drug Interactions

1) not to be taken with **aspirin** or **anticoagulants**[24] due to antithrombin activity of aesculin[2]

## HORSE RADISH

*Armoracia rusticana = Cochlearia armoracia*
fresh root
(meerrettich, grand raifort, raifort sauvage)

### Contraindications

1) **stomach ulcers** or **intestinal ulcers**[6] due to its stimulant effect on the gastric mucosa[5]

2) **kidney inflammation**[6] due to its strong diuretic effect[5]

3) **children** under age 4 due to potential gastrointestinal disturbances[6]

4) **pregnancy** due to its potential abortifacient effect[6]

## HORSETAIL

*\*Equisetum* spp. plant
(shave grass, scouring rush, bottle brush, paddock pipes, dutch rushes, pewterwort, schachtelhalm, zinnkraut, prele, pribe des champs, cola de caballo)

### Contraindications

1) **cardiovascular disease** and **high blood pressure**[2,24] though a study showed its hemostatic substance is not a vasoconstrictor and it has no effect on blood pressure when taken orally[11]

2) **vitamin $B_1$ deficiency** states due to thiaminase activity of plants[2,3]

### Drug Interactions

1) **digitalis** and its **cardiac glycosides** may become more toxic due to the loss of potassium from its diuretic effect[2,12]

2) causes breakdown of **thiamine**[2]

## HYSSOP

*Hyssopus officinalis* plant
(ysop, hysope)

### Contraindications

1) **pregnancy**[2] due to its emmenagogue[2,7,74] and abortifacient effects[2,74]

## IPECAC

*\*Cephalis ipecacuanha* root
(ipecacuanha)

### Contraindications

1) irritative or **corrosive poisonings** [1] prohibit its use as an emetic due to re-exposure of esophageal tissue to corrosives

2) **pregnancy**[2] since its alkaloid component (emetine) is a uterine stimulant in animal uteri[2,74]

3) organic **heart disease**[1,2] due to its depressive effect on the heart[2]

## JAMAICA DOGWOOD

*\*Piscidia erythrina* bark

### Contraindications

1) in **children** and **elderly**[1] due to potent neural depressant effect[2,3] caused by rotenone and isoflavones (ichthynone, piscidone, and piscerythrone)[3]

## JOE-PYE WEED

*\*Eupatorium purpureum* root
(gravel root, queen of the meadow, kidney root, purple boneset, trumpet weed)

## Contraindications

1) **excessive use** or **prolonged use** due to its hepatotoxic pyrrolizidine alkaloid content[6]

## JUNIPER

*Juniperus communis* berries
(common juniper, germeiner wacholder, wacholderbeeren, genevrier commun, genevieve, baies de genievre, enebro, ginepro)

## Contraindications

1) **kidney inflammation**[1,4,6,7,24] and **kidney infection**[6] due to irritation of the kidneys[2,6,24] by hydrocarbon volatile oil components (pinenes and cadinene) with frequent use or large doses[2,6]

2) **pregnancy**[1,2,4,6,7,24] due to its emmenogogue effect[2,24,74] and the abortifacient effect of its volatile oil[74] from urinary tract irritation leading to reflex uterine stimulation[4]

3) **prolonged use** for over 4 weeks due to potential for renal damage[6]

## KAVA-KAVA

*Piper methysticum* root
(kava, intoxicating long pepper, ava pepper shrub, rauschpfeffer)

## Contraindications

1) **pregnancy**[6] possibly due to loss of uterine tone[22]

2) **nursing mothers**[6] due to possible passage of pyrones into milk

3) **endogenous depression**[6] due to the sedative activity of its pyrones (kawain, methysticin, yangonin, and derivatives)[22]

### Drug Interactions

1) CNS **depressants**[6] enhanced due to sedative and muscle-relaxant effects of kava pyrones[22]

2) hypnotic effect of **alcohol** is enhanced by kava,[23] which can also impact driving ability[6]

## KHELLA

*Ammi visnaga* fruit

(toothpick ammi, bischofskraut, zahnstocher-ammei, herbe au cure-dents)

### Contraindications

1) **pregnancy** due to its emmenagogue effect and the uterine stimulant activity of its constituent khellin[3,74]

2) excessive **ultraviolet light** or **solarium therapy** due to the photosensitizing effect of its constituent khellin[3]

### Drug Interactions

1) decreases the toxicity of the cardiac glycoside **digitoxin** due to the coronary vasodilator and anti-arrhythmic effects[3]

## KNOT GRASS

*Polygonum aviculare* plant

(knotweed, beggarweed, bird knotgrass, birdweed, cow grass, common knotweed, crawlgrass, doorweed, ninety-knot, pigweed, vogelknoterich, wegtritt, renouee des oiseaux, centinode, sanguinaria jayor)

### Contraindications

1) **pregnancy** due to its abortifacient effect[2,74]

## LAVENDER

*Lavandula officinalis = Lavandula vera =
Lavandula angustifolia* flowers
(echter lavendel, lavande commun, espliego,
lavanda, spigo, nardo )

### Contraindications
1) **pregnancy** due to its emmenagogue effect[2]

## LEPTANDRA

*\*Veronicastrum virginicum = Veronica virginica*
root
(black root, Culver's root, Beaumont root,
Bowman's root, Culver's physic, hini, oxadoddy,
physic root, purple leptandra, tall speedwell, tall
veronica, whorlywort)

### Contraindications
1) **gallstones, hardened stones, or bile duct
obstruction**[1] due to its cholagogue effect[5]
2) internal **hemorrhoids** or during **menstruation**[1]
due to its cathartic effect[5]
3) threatened **miscarriage**[1] due to its abortifacient
activity when fresh[2,5]
4) **pregnancy**[1,2] due to its teratogenic effect[1] and
abortifacient activity when fresh[2,5]

## LICORICE

*\*Glycyrrhiza glabra* root
(sweet licorice, sweet wood, sweetwort, liquorice,
lakritze, sutholz, sussholz, bois doux, reglisse,
orozuz)

### Contraindications
1) severe **kidney insufficiency**[6] or **high blood
pressure** due to the sodium and fluid retention

from pseudoaldosteronism caused by its saponin (glycyrrhizin)[2,4,6]

2) **low blood potassium** or **cardiac disease**[4] due to increased potassium excretion from kidneys[4]

3) **prolonged use** for more than 4-6 weeks due to the mineral corticoid effects resulting in hypertension, hypokalemia, and edema[4,6]

4) **pregnancy**[2,4,6] due to its emmenogogue effect[2,74] and phytoestrogen components[2]

5) **liver cirrhosis, bile stasis disorders**[4,6] or **chronic hepatitis**[6] due to its choleretic effects[4]

## Drug Interactions

1) potentiates the toxicity of **cardiac glycosides**[4,6] such as those in **digitalis**[2,4,24] due to potassium loss in urine[4,6]

2) increases potassium loss from **thiazide diuretics,** but should also not be used simultaneously with either **spironolactone** or **amiloride**[4]

3) not to be used with **corticoid** treatment since glycyrrhizin interfers with 5β-reductase breakdown of corticosteroids, thus prolonging its biological half-life[21]

## LIFE ROOT

*Senecio aureus* plant
(ragwort, cocash weed, coughweed, golden ragwort, grundy swallow, squaw weed)

## Contraindications

1) **pregnancy** due to its emmenagogue,[2,7] oxytocic,[10] and teratogenic effects[2] and content of hepatotoxic pyrrolizidine alkaloids (senecine, senecifoline)[2,24,38]

2) **nursing mothers** due to excretion of hepatotoxic pyrrolizidine alkaloids into milk[38]

## LOBELIA

*Lobelia inflata* plant or seeds
(Indian tobacco, emetic herb, emetic weed,
gagroot, vomitroot, vomitwort, wild tobacco)

### Contraindications

1) **nervous prostration, shock,** or **paralysis**[1] due
to secondary depressant effect on preganglionic
nicotinic receptors by the alkaloid (lobeline)
2) dyspnea from chronic **heart disease**[24] such as
an **enlarged heart** or **fatty heart, fluid around
heart,** enfeebled heart with **valvular
incompetence,** asthma of **cardiac
decompensation, cardiac sinus arrhythmia** or
**bundle branch block**[1] due to interference of
lobeline with the heart's neural conductivity[2,3]
3) **pneumonia** or **fluid around lungs** as pleural
effusion,[1] possibly due to the respiratory stimulant
effect of lobeline[3]
4) **high blood pressure**[1] due to the α-adrenergic
hypertensive effects of lobeline[3]
5) **low vitality** or as an emetic to **children** or **the
elderly**[1] due to the depressive effect of lobeline[3]
6) **pregnancy**[24] possibly because it relaxes the
uterine os and perineal musculature[5]
7) **tobacco sensitivity**[24] due to the similarity of
lobeline to nicotine[2,3]

## LOVAGE

*Levisticum officinale = Ligusticum levisticum* root
(European lovage, lavose, sea parsley, liebstockel,
liveche)

### Contraindications

1) acute **kidney inflammation** or **urinary tract
inflammation** and **kidney insufficiency**[6,7] due to

its potential for causing kidney damage in excessive doses[7]

2) **pregnancy** due to its emmenagogue effect[7]

## MADDER

*Rubia tinctorum* root

(farberrote, krapp, garance)

### Contraindications

1) **pregnancy** due to its genotoxic[6] and emmenagogue effects[7]

2) **nursing mothers** due to its genotoxic effect[6]

## MA HUANG

*Ephedra sinica* = *Ephedra vulgaris* plant

(Chinese ephedra)

### Contraindications

1) **pregnancy**[2,20] due to its uterine stimulant action on animal uteri[2] associated with the alkaloids ephedrine and pseudoehedrine[74]

2) **anorexia**[2] due to the appetite suppressive effects of its alkaloids[29]

3) **insomnia**[2] due to its adrenergic stimulant effects[2]

4) **suicidal tendencies** due to the anxiety, tenseness, and apprehension caused by the sympathomimetic activity of ephedrine[2]

5) organic **heart disease** due to its adrenergic cardiac stimulant and arrhythmic effects[2,20]

6) **high blood pressure** due to the peripheral vasoconstrictive effects of its adrenergic ephedrine and pseudoephedrine components[2,20]

7) **diabetes**[20,30] due to the hyperglycemic action of ephedrine[30]

8) **excess thyroid** activity[20,29] due to the immediate increase in metabolic rate from its alkaloids[29] and the increased $T_3$ to $T_4$ ratio after four weeks of use of ephedrine[30]

9) **prostatic enlargement** with urinary retention[13,20] due to the alpha-adrenergic activity of the alkaloids that causes contraction of the bladder neck and prostate musculature[13]

10) **stimulant sensitivity** due to its central nervous system stimulation[20]

11) **stomach ulcers**[20] due to possible reduction of gastric secretion of protective mucus

12) **nursing mothers**[20] due to possible effects on sensitive infants

### Drug Interactions

1) increased thermogenesis and weight loss due to a reduction of body fat when ephedrine component is combined with **methylxanthines including theophylline**[18,19] and **caffeine**[18,19,20]

2) ephedrine can induce toxicity from **monoamine oxidase inhibitors (MAOI)**[20,46,47,48] due to increased release of noradrenaline by ephedrine[20,48] even after stopping MAOI medication and should be avoided for 2 weeks after stopping the MAOI[47]

## MALE FERN

*Dryopteris filix-mas* rhizome
(aspidium, bear's paw root, knotty brake, sweet brake, farnkraut, fongere, marginal shield-fern)

### Contraindications

1) **pregnancy** due to its abortifacient effect[2]

2) **anemia** or in **elderly** or **debilitated subjects** due to the impaired respiration/circulation caused[2]

3) **stomach ulcers** and **intestinal ulcers** due to the mucosal irritants in the oleoresin (filmaron and filicic acid)[2]

4) **heart disorders** due to its cardiac depressive effects[2]

5) **kidney insufficiency** or **liver disorders** due to the albuminuria and bilirubinuria it may cause[2]

## MANNA-ASH

*Fraxinus ornus* stem exudate

(flowering ash, flake manna, manna-esche, frene a la manne, orne a manne)

### Contraindications

1) **intestinal obstruction** due to its laxative effect[6]

## MARJORAM

*Origanum marjorana* = *Origanum hortensis* plant

(sweet marjoram, knotted marjoram, garden marjoram, majoran, marjolaine, origan marjolaine, mejorana, maggiorana)

### Contraindications

1) **pregnancy** due to its emmenagogue effect[2]

## MARSHMALLOW

*Althaea officinalis* root

(mortification root, sweet weed, wymote, eibischwurzel, malve, apothekerstockmalve, witte malve, guimauve, malvavisco, malvavisco, malvacioni, bismalva, buonvischio, hitmi, kitmi, gul hatem)

### Drug Interactions

1) absorption of **oral drugs** taken simultaneously may be delayed[6]

## MARSH TEA

*Ledum palustre* plant
(marsh cistus, moth herb, James' tea, Labrador tea,
swamp tea, wild rosemary, sumpfporst, romarin
sauvage)

### Contraindications

1) **pregnancy**[2,6] due to its abortifacient effect,
probably secondary to potent irritation by essential
oil of the urinary tract,[6] and its uterine stimulant
action in animal uteri[2,74]

## MASTERWORT

*Heracleum lanatum* plant
(cow parsnip, cow cabbage, hogweed, madnep,
woolly parsnip, youthwort)

### Contraindications

1) **pregnancy** due to its emmenagogue effect[2]

## MAYAPPLE

*Podophyllum peltatum* root/rhizome
(American mandrake, duck's foot, ground lemon,
hog apple, Indian apple, raccoon berry, wild
lemon, wild mandrake, entenfut, podophylle
americain)

### Contraindications

1) **gallstones**[1] due to the cholagogue effect of its
podophyllin resin on bile secretion[5]
2) **intestinal obstruction**[1] due to the profuse
cathartic action caused by its two peltatin
components[2,5]
3) **debilitated subjects**[1] due to its potent depleting
effect[1]

4) **pregnancy** due to the teratogenic[1,2,6,7,10] and feticidal effects of its podophyllotoxin and the peltatin components[2] (including the topical use of the resin)[8]

5) topical use of the resin **near the eye,**[8,24] in subjects with **diabetes,** or others with poor circulation, on **moles, birthmarks,** or **inflamed** or **irritated warts** since permanent damage can result due to the escharotic effects, or **over large areas** because of toxicity from absorption[8]

### Drug Interactions

1) common table **salt** increases its purgative power[2,5]

2) **lobelia, ipecac, leptandra, hyoscyamus** or **belladonna** render its effect milder[5]

## MEADOWSWEET

*Filipendula ulmaria = Spiraea ulmaria* flowers (bridewort, dolloff, meadsweet, meadow queen, meadow-wort, pride of the meadow, queen of the meadow, madesut, spierblumen, reine des pres, ulmaire)

### Contraindications

1) **allergic hypersensitivity** to its salicylates[4,6,24]

## MILK THISTLE

*Silybum marianum = Carduus marianus* seeds (holy thistle, Marythistle, St. Mary's thistle, Mariendistel, chardon-Marie)

### Drug Interactions

1) helps prevent liver damage from hepatotoxins including **butyrophenones, phenothiazines,**[84] **acetaminophen, halothane, dilantin,** and **ethanol** due to membrane-stabilizing and antioxidant

effects of the flavonolignans (silybin, silydianin, silychristin)[3]

## MISTLETOE

*Viscum album* plant
(European mistletoe, all-heal, birdlime, devil's fuge, mistel, vogelmistel, leimmistel, hexenbesen, drudenfut, herbe de gui, muerdago)

### Contraindications
1) **pregnancy** due to the uterine stimulant action shown in animal uteri by its constituent tyramine[2,74]

## MOTHERWORT

*Leonurus cardiaca* plant
(lion's ear, lion's tail, Roman motherwort, throwwort, herzgespann, agripaume)

### Contraindications
1) **pregnancy**[2] due to its emmenogogue effect[7] and the uterine stimulant action of its constituents stachydrine and leonurine on animal uteri[2,74]

## MUGWORT

*Artemisia vulgaris* plant
(common mugwort, felon herb, sailor's tobacco, gemeiner beifut, armoise)

### Contraindications
1) **pregnancy** due to its emmenagogue and abortifacient effects[2,6,74] and uterine stimulant action on animal uteri[2,74] associated with its major volatile constituent (thujone)[15]

## MUSTARD

*Brassica nigra* seed
(black mustard, echter kohl, moutarde noir,
mostaza, senape, mostarda)

### Contraindications

1) **irritative poisoning** or **corrosive poisonings**[1] disallows its internal use as an emetic due to the re-exposure of esophageal tissue to corrosives[2]

2) **stomach inflammation** or **intestinal inflammation** due to the irritation cause by allyl isothiocyanate release[2,5]

3) **pregnancy**[1,2] due to its potential abortifacient effect when taken in large amounts[2,74]

4) **externally over unprotected skin**[2,7] or applied **for a long time**[5,7] due to blistering and ulceration caused by isothiocyanate in the volatile oil[2,5,7]

## MYRRH

*Commiphora myrrha = Commiphora molmol*
gum-resin
(gum myrrh, myrrhe)

### Contraindications

1) acute, **internal inflammation**[1,5] since large doses can cause gastric burning[5]

2) **fever**[1,5] since it augments the heat of the body[5]

3) **arterial agitation** or excitement since large doses can accelerate the pulse[5]

4) **pregnancy**[2] due to its emmenagogue[2,5,74] and abortifacient effects[2,74]

### Drug Interactions

1) precipitates when mixed with **water** and adheres to the container[9]

## NIGHT-BLOOMING CEREUS
*Selenicereus grandiflorus* = *Cactus grandiflorus*
fresh stems
(cactus, large-flowered cactus, sweet-scented
cactus, vanilla cactus, cereus grand, konigin der
nacht, ciege a grandes fleurs)

**Contraindications**
1) **high blood pressure** or **heart over-activity**[1]
due to cardiac-stimulating effect[3]

## NUTMEG
*Myristica fragrans* seeds
(muskatbaum, muscadier)

**Contraindications**
1) **pregnancy** due to its potential abortifacient
effect[2,6,10,74] in toxic doses[6]

**Drug Interactions**
1) may potentiate **psychoactive drugs** due to its
mild monoamine oxidase inhibiting action[10]

## OAK
*Quercus* spp. bark
(eicherinde, chene, gravelier, encina)

**Contraindications**
1) **externally on skin damage over a large area**
due to absorption of tannins[4]

**Drug Interactions**
1) **alkaloids** and other **basic drugs** may have
reduced absorption[4,6] due to precipitation by the
tannins[2,9]

## OAT

Avena sativa immature seed

(hafer, avoine, avena)

### Drug Interactions

1) antagonizes the antinociceptive effect of **morphine**[54]

2) antagonizes the pressor reponse to **nicotine**[54]

## OLIVE

Olea europaea oil

(olivenbaum, olivier)

### Contraindications

1) **locally on the eye** due to its irritating effect on the surface[1]

2) **bile stones** due to risk of inducing biliary colic[6] by its cholagogue effect[7]

## PAPAYA

Carica papaya latex from unripe fruit

(custard apple, melon tree, pawpaw, melonenbaum, papayer)

### Contraindications

1) **allergic hypersensitivity** to chymopapain occurring in 1% of patients can lead to anaphylaxis[24]

## PAREIRA

Chondodendron tomentosum root

(pareira brava)

### Contraindications

1) **pregnancy** due to its emmenagogue effect[24]

## PARSLEY

*Petroselinum sativum* = *Apium petroselinum* fruit
(common parsley, garden parsley, rock parsley,
gartenpetersilie, petersilie, persil)

### Contraindications

1) **pregnancy**[2,6,7] due to the emmenogogue
effect[2,7,74] and animal uterine stimulant action of its
volatile oil (apiole)[2,74]

2) **kidney inflammation**[6,7] due to the toxicity of
the essential oil component apiole[6]

## PASSION FLOWER

*Passiflora incarnata* leaves
(Maypops, passion vine, purple passion flower,
passionblume, fleischfarbige passionsblume, fleur
de la passion, passiflore)

### Contraindications

1) **pregnancy** due to the uterine stimulant action
of its alkaloid content (harman)[2,74] and its content
of a cyanogenic glycoside (gynocardin)[3]

### Drug Interactions

1) the active sedative component maltol increases
sleeping time induced by **hexobarbital**[60]

## PEACH PIT

*Prunus persica* seeds

### Contraindications

1) **pregnancy** due to its emmenagogue and
abortifacient effects[2,74] and its content of a
cyanogenic glycoside (amygdalin)[2,24]

## PENNYROYAL

*Hedeoma pulegioides* plant
(American pennyroyal, mock pennyroyal,
mosquito plant, squaw balm, squawmint,
tickweed)

### Contraindications

1) **pregnancy** due to the emmengogue and
abortifacient effects[2,7,74] associated with reflexive
uterine stimulation from the urinary tract irritation
by its volatile oil components (pulegone)[2]

2) **kidney disease** due to irritation of the kidneys
by the volatile oil[2]

## PEONY

*Paeonia officinalis* root
(common peony, echte pfingstrose, peone, pivoine
officinale)

### Contraindications

1) **pregnancy** due to its emmenagogue effect[2,74]

## PEPPERMINT

*Mentha piperita* leaves
(brandy mint, lamb mint, pfefferminz, katzenkraut,
frauenmussatze, grune rossmunze, menthe
anglaise, menthe poivree, feuilles de menthe,
menthe de notre dame, menthe verte, menta
piperita, erba Santa Maria, mente vere)

### Contraindications

1) **pregnancy** due to its emmenagogue effect[2,74]
2) **gallstones** due to its choleretic activity[4]
3) **hiatal hernia**[24] due to its relaxing effect on the
lower esophageal sphincter[25]

## PERIWINKLE

*Vinca rosea* plant
(sinngrun, pervenche, pervinca, pervince,
maagdepalm, kucuk)

**Contraindications**
1) **pregnancy** due to its teratogenic effects[2]

## PERUVIAN BALSAM

*Myroxylon pereirae* oleoresin of fruit
(balsam of Peru)

**Contraindications**
1) **allergic hypersensitivity**[6] due to its cinnamein
content[10]
2) **extended use** of more than 1 week or **excessive
concentration** over 10% when applied **externally**
to large surfaces[6] due to its potential for allergic
skin reactions[6,10]

## PINE

*Pinus* spp. needles
(common pine, fichtensprossen, pin, pino)

**Contraindications**
1) **pregnancy** due to potential abortifacient
effects[6]

## PLEURISY ROOT

*Asclepias tuberosa* root
(butterfly weed, Canada root, flux root, orange
swallow-wort, tuber root, white root, wind root)

**Contraindications**
1) **pregnancy** due to the uterine stimulant action
on animal uteri[2,72,74] and its estrogenic activity[72]

## POMEGRANATE

*Punica granatum* root bark

### Contraindications

1) **pregnancy** due to its emmenogogue effect and uterine stimulation action on animal uteri[2,74]

## PRICKLY ASH

*Xanthoxylum americanum* = *Zanthoxylum americanum* bark

(toothache bush, toothache tree, yellow wood)

### Contraindications

1) acute **stomach ulcers** and/or **intestinal ulcers**[1] due to its stimulating gastrointestinal mucosal secretions[5]
2) **stomach inflammation** or **intestinal inflammation**[1] due to its mucosal stimulation[5]
3) **pregnancy**[24] due to its emmengogoue effect[5]
4) **nursing mothers** probably since it can irritate the stomach[24]

## PRIMROSE

*Primula veris* = *Primula officinalis* flowers

(butter rose, English cowslip, primel, schlusselblume, primevere, primavera)

### Contraindications

1) **allergic hypersensitivity** due to rare contact allergy[6,7]

## PSYLLIUM

*Plantago psyllium* = *Plantago afra; Plantago ovata* = *Plantago ispaghula* seed

(fleaseed, psyllion, psyllios, strauchwegerich, plantain des sables, plantain pucier, blond psyllium, Indian plantago, ispaghula, spogel seed, Indisches psyllium, ispaghul)

## Contraindications

1) **esophageal stenosis** and **abnormal intestinal narrowing or**[4,6] **bowel obstruction**[24] due to the bulk forming effect which may cause, or further complicate, impaction[4]

2) difficult-to-control **diabetes** since insulin need may be reduced[4,6]

## Drug Interactions

1) reduced absorption of **oral drugs**[4,6] such as **lithium** salts[40]

2) **insulin** dosage may need reduction due to slowing of dietary carbohydrate absorption[4]

## PULSATILLA

*Anemone pulsatilla* = *Pulsatilla vulgaris* plant (pasque flower, wind flower, meadow anemone, meadow windflower, passe flower, Easter flower, kuchenschelle)

## Contraindications

1) **pregnancy**[2,6] due to its uterine stimulant action on animal uteri[2,74]

2) **nursing mothers**[24] because of its gastrointestinal irritant effect[2]

## QUEEN ANN'S LACE

*Daucus carota* seeds
(wild carrot, beesnest plant, bird's nest root, karotte, mohrrube, carotte)

**Contraindications**

1) **pregnancy** due to its emmenagogue and abortifacient effects and its uterine stimulant action on animal uteri[.2,74]

## RASPBERRY

*Rubus idaeus* leaves

(garden raspberry, European red raspberry, himbeere, framboisier)

**Contraindications**

1) **pregnancy with a history of rapid labor**[1,3] due to its uterine stimulant activity, as well as its having antigonadotropic activity[3]

## RHUBARB

*Rheum palmatum* root

(Chinese rhubarb, turkey rhubarb, rhabarber, rhubarbe de Chine, ruibarbo)

**Contraindications**

1) **pregnancy**[1,2,4,24] due to uterine stimulant action in animal uteri[.2,74]

2) **children** under age twelve due to depletion of water and electrolytes[6]

3) **fever** or **intestinal inflammatory diseases**[1,6] such as **Crohn's disease** and **ulcerative colitis** due to the irritating effects of the anthroquinone derivatives (rhein, emodin, aloe-emodin)[6]

4) **intestinal obstruction**[6] due to the cathartic effect of its anthranoid components (rhein, sennosides)[4,5,6]

5) **extended use** for more than 8 - 10 days due to pathological alterations to the colon smooth muscles and myenteric plexi[6]

6) **abdominal pain** of unknown origin[6] due to possible rupture from contraction of inflamed viscus such as the appendix

7) **nursing mothers**[6,24] due to passage of the anthraquinones into the milk[6]

8) **kidney disease**[24] since dehydration induced by laxatives may aggrevate nephropathy[6]

9) **hemorrhoids**[24] due to the potential for inducing or aggravating hemorrhoidal thrombosis and/or prolapsis[6]

### Drug Interactions

1) reduced absorption of **oral drugs** due to decreases bowel transit time[6]

2) overuse or misuse can cause potassium loss leading to increased toxicity of **cardiac glycosides**[4,6] such as those in *Adonis, Convallaria, Urginea,*[2,6] *Helleborus, Strophanthus,* and *Digitalis*[2]

3) aggravates potassium loss from use of **diuretics**[6]

## ROSEMARY

*Rosmarinus officinalis* leaves

(rosmarin, incensier, romero, rosmarino, ramerino)

### Contraindications

1) **pregnancy**[4,6] due to its emmenagogue effect[7] from toxic amounts of components of the essential oil[4]

## RUE

*Ruta graveolens* leaves and unripe fruit

(common rue, garden rue, German rue, herb-of-grace, raute, ruda)

### Contraindications

1) **pregnancy**[1,2,7] due to its emmenogogue[74,75] and abortifacient effects[10,74,75] and the uterine stimulant activity of its constituent skimmianine[2,74]

2) excessive exposure to **ultraviolet light** due to possible photodermatitis reaction[6]

## SAFFRON

*Crocus sativa* stigma and styles

(autumn crocus, Spanish saffron, safran)

### Contraindications

1) **pregnancy**[2,4] due to its emmenogogue[7,10] and abortifacient effects in toxic doses[2,4,6,74]

## SAGE

*Salvia officinalis* leaves

(garden sage, sawge, edelsalbei, salbei, sauge)

### Contraindications

1) **pregnancy** due to its emmenagogue[2,4,6,15,74] and abortifacient effects[74] associated with its volatile oil (thujone) content[2,4,6,15]

2) **prolonged use** due to possible epileptiform cramps[6]

## SANDALWOOD

*Santalum album* wood

(white sandalwood, white saunders, yellow sandalwood, sandelholz, weisser sandelbaum, santal blanc, sandalia, sandalo bianco, chaudana)

### Contraindications

1) **pregnancy** due to its abortifacient effect[2,74]

2) **kidney disease**[6] due to its diuretic effect[7]

3) **prolonged use** for more than 6 weeks[6] probably due to its volatile oil content[5,7]

## SASSAFRAS

*Sassafras albidum* bark
(ague tree, cinnamon wood, saxifrax, fenchelholz, bois odorant, sassafraso, lauro degl'Trocchesi)

### Contraindications
1) **pregnancy**[1,2] due to its emmenogogue effect[2,74]
2) **prolonged use** of forms (e.g., alcoholic extract) containing containing its essential oil (safrole) due to its toxic and hepatocarcinogenic effects[6]

## SAVIN

*Juniperus sabina* tops
(savine)

### Contraindications
1) general or local **inflammation**[1,5] due to irritation caused by the essential oil (sabinene and sabinyl acetate) from direct contact externally with the skin or internally on mucosa, resulting in gastroenteritis, hepatitis, pneumonitis and nephritis when taken in an oral overdose[6]
2) **pregnancy**[1,5] due to its abortifacient effect[5,6]

## SCOTCH BROOM

*Cytisus scoparius* = *Sarothamnus scoparius* tops
(broom, link, Irish broom, besenginster, genet a balai)

### Contraindications
1) **high blood pressure**[1,6] due to the cardiac stimulant activity of an alkaloid component (sparteine)[2,5,6]

2) acute **kidney disorders**[1] due to the diuretic
activity of its component scoparin[5]
3) **spleen** and **liver disorders**[1] based upon
empirical results
4) **pregnancy**[1,2] due to the abortifacient effect and
uterine stimulant activity of sparteine[74]

## Drug Interactions

1) **monoamine oxidase inhibitors** due to the high
content of tyramine[6]

## SENEGA

*Polygala senega* root
(milkwort, mountain flax, seneca root, rattlesnake
root, Seneca snakeroot, Senega snakeroot,
klapperschlangenwurzel)

## Contraindications

1) active **feverish conditions**[1] due to its CNS
depressant effect[2]
2) active **inflammation** due to its local stimulant
activity[5] and intestinal irritant effects[2]
3) **pregnancy** due to its uterine stimulant action on
animal uteri[.2,74]

## SENNA

*Cassia acutifolia* = *Cassia senna* leaves or pods
(locust plant, wild senna, Alexandrian senna,
Alexandriner-senna, sene d'Alexandrie, sene de
Khartoum )

## Contraindications

1) **intestinal obstruction**[4,6,24] due to stimulation of
peristalsis by its anthroquinones (sennosides)[4,6]
2) **stomach inflammation**[1,5] due to griping[5] and
**intestinal inflammatory diseases**[1,5,6] such as

ulcerative colitis and **Crohn's disease**[6] due to
irritation caused by anthroquinones[4]
3) **anal prolapse**[5] due to aggravation by enhancing
the bowel's expulsive force[4]
4) **hemorrhoids**[5] due to possible induction of
stenosis, thrombosis, and prolapse[6]
5) **pregnancy**[4] due to possible endometrial
stimulation[6,24] and passage of genotoxic aloe-
emodin across placenta[6]
6) **nursing mothers** due to passage of
anthroquinones into mother's milk[4,5,6]
7) **children** under age 12 due to water and
electrolyte loss[6]
8) **extended use** for more than 8-10 days[6,24] due to
decreased peristalsis from intestinal smooth
muscle damage[6]
9) **appendicitis** and **abdominal pain** whose cause
in unknown[24] due to possibly inducing a rupture
from contraction of the inflamed organ

## Drug Interactions

1) sennosides aggravate nephropathy from
**analgesics** associated with dehydration[6]
2) decrease absorption of **oral drugs** due to
decrease in bowel transit time[6]
3) overuse or misuse can cause potassium loss
leading to increased toxicity of **cardiac
glycosides**[4,6] such as those in *Adonis, Convallaria,
Urginea,*[2,6] *Helleborus, Strophanthus,* and
*Digitalis*[2]
4) aggravates loss of potassium associated with use
of **diuretics**[6]

## SHEPHERD'S PURSE

*Capsella bursa-pastoris* plant
(cocowort, pick-pocket, St. James' weed,
shepherd's heart, toywort, hirtentaschel, bourse a
pasteur, fleur de S. Jacques, bolsa de pastor, borsa
di pastore)

### Contraindications

1) **pregnancy** due to its emmenagogue[2,74] and
abortifacient effect and the uterine stimulant
action[2,7,74]

## SIBERIAN GINSENG

*Eleutherococcus senticosus* = *Acanthopanax
senticosus* root

(touch-me-not, devil's shrub, wild pepper,
eleuthero ginseng, devil's bush, taigawurzel,
eleutherocoque)

### Contraindications

1) **high blood pressure**[6] probably due to the
increased production of adrenalin in the adrenal
glands[3]

### Drug Interactions

1) increases effect of **hexobarbital**[3,6] due to
inhibition of its metabolic breakdown[3]
2) increases efficacy of **antibiotics** probably due to
enhancement of T-lymphocyte activity[3]

## ST. JOHN'S WORT

*Hypericum perforatum* plant
(amber, goatweed, Johnswort, Klamath weed,
Tipton weed, hardhay, hartheu, Johanniskraut,
blutkraut, herrgottsblut, walpurgiskraut,
hexenkraut, millepertuis)

## Contraindications

1) **pregnancy** due to its emmenagogue and abortifacient effects and its uterine stimulant action on animal uteri[2,3,74]

2) **ultraviolet light** or **solarium therapy** due to potential photosensitizing effects[4,6] if large doses of its hypericin component are used[4]

3) **endogenous depression**[24] when severe, since it has only been shown to be effective in mild or moderate forms of depression[95]

## Drug Interactions

1) **foods or drugs interacting with monoamine oxidase inhibitors** are contraindicated due to the inhibition of monoamine oxidase by xanthones[49] and a number of flavonoid components of St. Johns wort[50]

2) sleeping time of **narcotics** is enhanced and the effects of **reserpine** are antagonised[51]

## STINGING NETTLE

*Urtica* spp. plant
(nettle, common nettle, great stinging nettle, common stinging nettle, brennessel, hanfnessel, ortie, ortiga, ortica)

## Contraindications

1) **pregnancy** due to its emmenagogue and abortifacient effects when used in excessively large quantities, and the uterine stimulant action of its serotonin constituent on animal uteri[2,3,74]

## SWEET CLOVER

*Melilotus officinalis* plant
(yellow melilot, field melilot, hay flowers, king's
clover, yellow sweet clover, steinklee, honigklee,
mottenklee, barenklee, mallotenkraut, petit trefle
jaune, trefle des mouches, herbe aux puces,
couronne royale, melilot)

### Drug Interactions

1) **salicylates, acetaminophen,** and **bromelain**
due to potential hemorrhagic diathesis[2,31] from its
coumarin components[2,5,31]

## TANSY

*Tanacetum vulgare* leaves
(bitter buttons, hindheal, parsley fern)

### Contraindications

1) **pregnancy** due to the emmenagogue[2,7,15,74,75]
and abortifacient effect[2,7,15] from uterine stimulant
action caused by its volatile oil (thujone)[2,15,74]

## TEA

*Camellia sinensis* = *Thea sinensis* leaves
(black tea, green tea, oolong tea, Chinesischer tee,
theier)

### Contraindications

1) **kidney disorders** since the diuretic effect of
caffeine and theophylline increase the urinary
output[8]
2) **duodenal ulcers** due to increased gastric acid
secretion from caffeine[8]
3) **heart disorders** due to acute and/or excessive
caffeine consumption increasing heart rate and
causing arrhythmias[8]

4) **psychological disorders** since caffeine can aggravate depression or induce anxiety neurosis[8]

## Drug Interactions

1) **oral contraceptives** and **cimetidine** increase the effect of caffeine[8]

2) increased thermogenesis and weight loss due to a reduction of body fat when its caffeine and/or theophylline components are combined with **ephedrine**[18,19] as well as agitation, tremors, and insomnia[19]

3) excessive amounts of caffeine taken with **monoamine oxidase inhibitors** can cause a hypertensive crisis

## THYME

*Thymus* spp. leaves

(garden thyme, common thyme, echter thymian, romischer quendel, thym, tomillo, timo)

### Contraindications

1) **pregnancy**[2] due to its emmenagogue effect[2,74]

## TOBACCO

*Nicotiana tabacum* leaves

### Contraindications

1) **pregnancy** due to lower birth weight and size and higher risk of prematurity, miscarriage, and neurological impairment to the baby[2,81]

2) members of families with **heart disease** due to increasing their risk by three times[81]

3) **cancer** associated with tobacco use including lung, mouth, pharyngeal, laryngeal, esophageal, bladder, and pancreatic cancers due to continuing exacerbation[81]

4) tobacco **smoking-related diseases** including **ulcers, high blood pressure, diabetes,**

osteoporosis, blood clots in the legs, and
glaucoma due to possible exacerbation of existing
conditions[81]
5) prior to medical lab tests due to the many
changes and false positives induced by smoking[81]
6) regular and/or excessive toxin exposure due to
adverse combined effects of tobacco with carbon
monoxide, asbestos, particulate matter, heavy
metals, and other xenobiotics[81]
7) poor health due to lifestyle-related conditions
such as obesity, alcoholism, and lack of
exercise[81]
8) type A personality due to the increased risk of
heart disease[81]
9) prior to surgery due to the increased number of
complications from higher carbon monoxide levels
in the blood[81]

### Drug Interactions

1) decreases the blood levels of acetaminophen
and vitamin $B_{12}$[81]
2) speeds the elimination of amobarbital,
benzodiazepines, caffeine, heparin, pentazocine,
tricyclic antidepressants, and vitamin C[81]
3) phenylbutazoneestrogen, and theophylline are
metabolized more quickly[81]
4) furosemide, phenothiazines, propoxyphene,
and propanolol are less effective[81]
5) blocks action of cimetidine[81]
6) enhances the drug effects of glutethimide[81]
7) increases risk of clots, strokes and heart attack
in women over age 30 using oral contraceptives[81]

## TURMERIC

*Curcuma longa* = *Curcuma domestica* root
(Indian saffron, kurkumawurzelstock, gelbwurzel,
javanische, rhizome de curcuma, temoe-lawaq)

### Contraindications

1) **bile duct obstruction**[4,6] due to its cholagogue
activity[6] and the choleretic effect of its yellow
pigment (curcumin) (use with **gallstones** only after
consultation with a doctor)[4]

## VALERIAN

*\*Valeriana officinalis* root/rhizome
(fragrant valerian, all-heal, English valerian,
German valerian, wild valerian, heliotrope,
setwall, vandal root, Vermont valerian, baldrian,
herbe aux chats, valeriane, valeriana)

### Drug Interactions

1) volatile components increase sleeping time
induced by **pentobarbital**[52]

## WATERCRESS

*Nasturtium officinale* plant
(scurvy grass, tall nasturtium, brunnenkresse,
wasserkresse, cresson de Fontaine, cresson au
poulet, nasilord, berro di agua, crescione di fonte,
waterkres)

### Contraindications

1) **pregnancy**[2,7] due to its emmenagogue and
abortifacient effects[2,74]
2) **peptic ulcer**[6] since its juice can cause
inflammation of the stomach[7]
3) **kidney inflammation**[6] since excessive or
prolonged use can lead to kidney problems[7]

4) **children** under age 4 due to possible gastrointestinal upset[6]
5) **prolonged use** of more than 4 weeks due to potential kidney irritation[7]

## WILD CHERRY

*Prunus serotina* bark
(wild black cherry, black choke, choke cherry, rum cherry, kirschenstiele, tige de cerise, tallo de cereza)

### Contraindications

1) **pregnancy** due to its teratogenic effects and content of a cyanogenic glycoside (prunisin)[2]

## WILD GINGER

*Asarum canadensis* root/rhizome
(black snakeweed, Canada snakeroot, coltsfoot snakeroot, false coltsfoot, heart snakeroot, Indian ginger, southern snakeroot, Vermont snakeroot)

### Contraindications

1) **stomach inflammation** and/or **intestinal inflammation**[1,5] due to its spicey stimulant effects[5]
2) **pregnancy** due to its emmenogogue and abortifacient effects[10]

## WILD INDIGO

*Baptisia tinctoria* plant
(American indigo, horsefly weed, indigo broom, false indigo, yellow broom, yellow indigo)

### Contraindications

1) **hyperemia**[1] due to alkaloid (baptitoxine) and phenolic glycoside (baptin) gastrointestinal irritants[2]

## WILD MARJORAM

*Origanum vulgare* plant
(wilder majoran, marjolaine sauvage, origan)

### Contraindications

1) **pregnancy** due to its emmenagogue and abortifacient effects[2,74]

## WOOD SORREL

*Oxalis acetosella* plant
(common sorrel, cuckoo bread, green sauce, mountain sorrel, shamrock, sour trefoil, stubwort, white sorrel)

### Contraindications

1) **pregnancy** due to its emmenagogue effect[2,74]

## WORMSEED

*\*Chenopodium ambrosioides* seed
(feather geranium, goosefoot, Jerusalem oak, Jesuit tea, Mexican tea, American wormseed, wurmsamen)

### Contraindications

1) **pregnancy** due to the emmenogogue and abortifacient effects of the seed oil[2,74,75]
2) **stomach disease** or **intestinal disease**[2] since the seed oil acts as an irritant to the alimentary tract[2,3]
3) **heart disease**[2] since the seed oil acts as a cardiac depressant[2,3]
4) **liver disease** since the seed oil has toxic hepatic effects[2]
5) **repeated use** (more than once) of 1-3 cc of the seed oil in a one-week period[3]
6) use of seed oil alone in the **undernourished, in debilitated subjects,** or **in very young children**[3]

7) **kidney disease** since the seed oil has renal toxic effects[2,3]

## WORMWOOD

*Artemisia absinthium* tops and leaves
(wermut, meifuss, absinthe, armoise commune, ajenjo, zona diri Johannes, artemisa comun, erba di San Giovanni)

### Contraindications

1) **pregnancy** due to its emmenagogue[2,74] and abortifacient effects[15,74] and the uterine stimulant action on animal uteri by its thujone content[2,15]
2) **stomach ulcers** or **intestinal ulcers**[6] due to irritation of the stomach and stimulation of the GI tract[5]

## YARROW

*Achillea millefolium* plant
(milfoil, noble yarrow, nosebleed, sanguinary, soldier's woundwort, thousandleaf, gemeine schafgarbe, tausendaugbraum, achilee, herbe aux charpentiers, millefeuille, milefolio, millegoglie, erba da falegname, erba da carpentieri, civan percemi, roga mari, birangasifa)

### Contraindications

1) **pregnancy** due to its emmenogogue and abortifacient effects[2,74] if the essential oil (with its thujone content) is used[2,15]
2) **allergic hypersensitivity** to yarrow or other Asteracea (arnica, calendula, chamomile)[4] based on sesquiterpene lactone content[6]

## YELLOW CEDAR

*Thuja occidentalis* leaves
(arborvitae, tree of life, white cedar,
abendlandischer lebensbaum, thuya)

### Contraindications

1) **pregnancy**[2] due to its emmenogogue[7] and
abortifacient effects[2,15,74] and the uterine stimulant
activity[74] caused by its volatile oil (thujone)[2,15]

## YERBA MANSA

*Anemopsis californica* roots and rhizomes
(swamp root, lizard's tail, hierba del manso,
babisa, hoja de babisa, ch'-ponip, vavish, nupitchi,
comaanal)

### Drug Interactions

1) sedative effect of the roots caused by the
volatile component methyleugenol[53] potentiates
the hypnotic action of **pentobarbital,
thiopental,**[68] and **hexobarbital**[69] and enhances the
central depressant effect of **chlorpromazine**[68]

## YOHIMBE

*Pausinystalia yohimbe = Corynanthe yohimbe*
bark

### Contraindications

1) **schizophrenia** since psychotic episodes can be
induced[76]
2) bipolar **depression** since yohimbine may elicit
manic-like symptoms[77] or suicidal tendencies[76]
3) **allergic hypersensitivity** to yohimbe due to
possible development of dermititis, acute renal
failure, and lupus-like syndrome[78]

4) **anxiety** can be exacerbated and **high blood pressure** increased due to its major active alkaloid (yohimbine)[76,77,79]

5) **liver disease** or **kidney disease** due to antidiuresis and the normally rapid metabolism and elimination of its potent alkaloid yohimbine[2,80]

6) **pregnancy** or **prolonged use** due to a lack of teratolgy and long-term toxicological and carcinogenicity studies of its potent alkaloids[80]

## Drug Interactions

1) hypertension may occur with yohimbine and **tricyclic antidepressants**[77] such as **imipramine**[76]

2) toxicity of yohimbine due to its $\alpha_2$-adrenoceptor antagonism is increased by **phenothiazines**[77] such as **chlorpromazine**[79]

3) reversal of hypotensive effects of **clonidine** and similar **antihypertensives** due to yohimbine's $\alpha$-adrenergic antagonism[77]

4) anxiety induced by yohimbine was blocked by **reserpine** and hypertension induced by it was reduced by **reserpine, atropine, and amobarbital**[79]

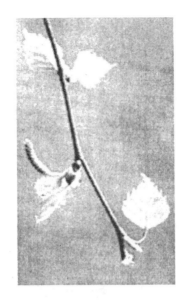

## APPENDICES

---

### Appendix A

### HERBS TO BE USED WITH CAUTION

### Appendix B

### HERB/DRUG INTERACTIONS

### Appendix C

### HERBS CONTRAINDICATED FOR MOTHERS

# Appendix A

# HERBS TO BE USED
# WITH CAUTION

## A.1 Due To Potential Allergic Response

### Section A.1.1 Aster Relatives

While an allergic response is theoretically possible with all plants or any substance, particular species have more commonly elicited an allergic hypersensitivity reaction.

Certain medicinal plants related to ragweed in the aster family (Asteraceae, formerly known as Compositae) may induce a cross-sensitivity resulting in contact dermatitis or other allergic effects, probably due to their content of certain sesquiterpene lactones. Allergic sensitivity to one of these plants may result in a similar sensitivity to the others in this list.

(Based on references 3, 4, 6, 10, 63, and 64.)

Arnica flowers *(*Arnica montana*)
Artichoke leaves (*Cynara scolymus*)
Blessed thistle (*Cnicus benedictus*)
Boneset (*Eupatorium perfoliatum*)
Burdock (*Arctium lappa*)
Camomile (*Anthemis cotula*)
Canada fleabane plant (*Erigeron canadensis*)
Chamomile, German flowers (*Matricaria recutita*)
Chamomile, Roman flowers (*Anthemis nobilis*)
Chicory root (*Cichorium intybus*)
Dandelion leaves and root (*Taraxacum officinale*)
Elecampane root (*Inula helenium*)

---

\* Denotes herbs in this appendix having other side effects when taken in excessive doses.

Goldenrod tops (*Solidago virgaurea*)
Hemp agrimony *(*Eupatorium cannabinum*)
Mugwort (*Artemisia vulgaris*)
Sagebrush leaves and tops (*Artemisia* spp.)
Spiny clot-bur plant (*Xanthium spinosum*)
Tansy tops *(*Tanacetum vulgare*)
Wormwood *(*Artemisia absinthium*)
Yarrow leaves and flowers (*Achillea millefolium*)

### Section A.1.2    Salicylates

Several genera of the **Salicaceae (#)** and individual plants of other families contain salicylates that may induce idiosyncratic reactions in susceptible individuals.
(Based on references 3, 4, 6, and 10.)

Black cohosh rhizome *(*Cimicifuga racemosa*)
Meadowsweet flower (*Filipendula ulmaria* = *Spiraea ulmaria*)
Poplar bark and/or buds (*Populus* spp.)#
Sweet birch bark (*Betula lenta*)
Willow bark (*Salix* spp.)#
Wintergreen leaves *(*Gaultheria procumbens*)

## A.2    Due To Phototoxic Effect

Certain medicinal plants of the Carrot family (Apiaceae, formerly known as Umbelliferae) can cause a photodermatitis in humans from sensitization of the skin to ultraviolet light due to their furanocoumarins which are similar in structure to psoralen. Furanocoumarins and components from plants of **non-Apiaceae families (#)** can act as photosensitizers. Use of plants containing any of these phototoxic components should be avoided during excessive periods in sunlight or while undergoing cosmetic or therapeutic ultraviolet light exposure, especially when 8-methoxypsoralen is being taken concurrently.
(Based on references 3, 4, 6, and 10.)

Angelica root (*Angelica* spp.)
Buttercup plant *(*Ranunculus* spp.)#
Celery (*Apium graveolens*)
Dill (*Anethum graveolens*)
Fennel (*Foeniculum vulgare*)

Khella fruit *(*Ammi visnaga*)
Lomatium root (*Lomatium dissectum*)
Masterwort (*Heracleum lanatum*)
Parsley (*Petroselinum sativum*)
Queen Ann's lace (*Daucus carota*)
Rue leaves *(*Ruta graveolens*)#
St. John's wort leaves and tops (*Hypericum perforatum*)#

## A.3   In Acute Inflammation Of The Urinary Tract

Plants containing volatile oils that are partially or primarily excreted through the kidneys have traditionally been used in treating urinary tract infections due to their antimicrobial activity. However, when the renal or mucosal tissue of the urinary tract are acutely inflamed, the irritant properties of these volatile substances can further aggravate kidney inflammation and urinary tract discomfort. Overdose or overuse of plants containing volatile constituents can even cause urinary tract inflammation when it does not already exist. Unless appropriate steps are taken to relieve, protect, or prevent the local inflammation, the use of plant remedies irritating to the urinary tract should be avoided.
(Based on references 1, 2, 5, and 7.)

Asparagus shoots (*Asparagus officinalis*)
Buchu leaves *(*Barosma betulina*)
Celery seed (*Apium graveolens*)
Cinnamon bark (*Cinnamomum zeylanicum*)
Copaiba oleoresin (*Copaiba langsdorffii*)
Cubeb unripe fruit *(*Piper cubeba*)
Dill seed (*Anethum graveolens*)
Eucalyptus leaves *(*Eucalyptus* spp.)
Fragrant sumach root bark (*Rhus aromatica*)
Juniper berries *(*Juniperus* spp.)
Parsley fruit *(*Petroselinum sativum*)
Pennyroyal leaves *(*Hedeoma pulegioides*)
Rue leaves *(*Ruta graveolens*)
Sandalwood bark (*Santalum album*)
Sassafras bark *(*Sassafras albidum*)
Thyme leaves *(*Thymus* spp.)
Yellow cedar leaves *(*Thuja occidentalis*)
Yerba mansa root/rhizome (*Anemopsis californica*)

# Appendix B

# HERB/DRUG INTERACTIONS

## B.1  Inhibiting Intestinal Absorption Of Medicines

### Section B.1.1  Hydrocolloidal Fibers

Plant parts or products containing water-soluble, hydrocolloidal fiber extracted in warm or cool water may slow absorption of oral drugs and reduce serum nutrient levels. This action results when these types of fiber are taken with medicine or food because of a resulting increased viscosity and delayed gastric emptying. These gums and mucilages are generally insoluble in alcohol.
(Based on references 4, 42, 43, 44, 61, and 62.)

Acacia tree exudate (e.g., *Acacia senegal*)
Agar powder, granules, flakes, or strips from certain red algae (e.g., *Gelidium cartilagineum, Gracilaria confervoides*)
Alginate powder from certain brown algae (e.g., *Macrocystis pyrifera*)
Aloe gel (*Aloe vera*)
Carrageenan gum from certain red algae (e.g., *Gigartina mamillosa*)
Fenugreek seed (*Trigonella foenum-graecum*)
Flax seed or meal remaining after expression of the linseed oil (*Linum usitatissimum*)
Furcellaran extract from a red algae (*Furcellaria fastigiata*)
Ghatti gum tree exudate (*Anogeissus latifolia*)
Guar gum seed endosperm (*Cyamopsis* spp.)
Iceland moss lichen (*Cetraria islandica*)
Irish moss red algae (*Chondrus crispus*)
Karaya gum tree exudate (e.g., *Sterculia uren, Cochlospermum gossypium*)
Konjac powder- glucomannan from tubers (*Amorphophallus konjac*)

---

* Denotes herbs in this appendix having other side effects when taken alone in excessive doses.

Locust bean gum - endosperm from seeds of carob tree (*Ceratonia siliqua*)
Marshmallow root (*Althaea officinalis*)
Oat seed β-glucans (*Avena sativa*)
Okra fruit (*Hibiscus esculentus*)
Pectin powder from apple pomace (*Malus domestica*) and citrus peels (e.g., *Citrus limon*)
Psyllium seed husks (*Plantago psyllium, Plantago ovata*)
Quince seed (*Cydonia vulgaris*)
Slippery elm bark (*Ulmus fulva*)
Tragacanth gummy exudate (*Astragalus gummifer*)

### Section B.1.2    Tannins and Salicylates

Plants and their parts which yield tannins when extracted by hot water can precipitate alkaloids in medicinal plants (e.g., *Atropa belladonna, Lobelia inflata*), alkaloidal drugs (e.g., ephedrine, colchicine), proteins (e.g., albumin), and metals (e.g., iron, copper) thereby slowing, reducing or blocking their absorption. Tannin content percentages are given when known. The alkaloidal precipitates are generally soluble in mixtures containing over 15-40% alcohol. Tannins will not precipitate low concentrations of alkaloidal salts in the presence of many of the gums listed above in Section B.1.1.

Alkaloids can also be precipitated by salicylates. (See Appendix A, Section A.1.2, for a listing of plants that contain salicylates.)

(Based on references 2, 7, and 9.)

Alder bark (*Alnus* spp.)
Alum root (*Heuchera americana*) 9-20%
Bayberry bark (*Myrica cerifera*)
Bearberry leaves (*Arctostaphylos uva-ursi*) 17-22%
Betelnut *(Areca catechu*) 11-26%
Bistort rhizome (*Polygonum bistorta*) 15-21%
Black walnut leaves, bark and rinds extract *(Juglans nigra*) 45%
Blackberry root bark (*Rubus villosus*) 10-13%
Catechu wood extract (*Acacia catechu*) 22-50%
Chestnut leaves (*Castanea dentata*) 9%
Cranesbill rhizome (*Geranium maculatum*) 10-25%
Douglas fir bark (*Pseudotsuga taxifolia*)
French rose petals (*Rosa gallica*) 5%
Gambir leaf and shoot extract (*Uncaria gambier*) 22-50%
Hemlock spruce bark (*Tsuga canadensis*)

Kino inspissated juice (*Pterocarpus marsupium*) 30-80%
Logwoood heartwood (*Hematoxylon campechianum*) 12%
Mountain laurel leaves (*Kalmia latifolia*)
Oak leaf galls (*Quercus infectoria*) 40-70%
Persimmon bark and unripe fruit (*Diospyros virginiana*)
Pomegranate rind (*Punica granatum*) 30%
Raspberry leaves (*Rubus idaeus*) 13-15%
Red pine bark (*Pinus resinosa*)
Red root dried bark (*Ceanothus americanus*) 10%
Rhatany root (*Krameria triandra*) 8-20%
Sumac leaves and fruit (*Rhus glabra*) 6-27%
Tanner's dock root (*Rumex hymenosepalus*) 9-32%
Tea leaves (*Camellia sinensis*) 9-13%
Tormentil root (*Potentilla tormentilla*)
White oak bark (*Quercus alba*) 6-11%
Witchhazel leaves (*Hamamelis virginiana*) 8-11%

## B.2    Potentiating Cardiotonic Medicines

### Section B.2.1    Herbal Cardiotonics

Some plants contain steroidal cardiac glycosides similar to those contained in or derived from digitalis. By their additive effects, such glycosides can produce cardiac toxicity when used with digitalis glycosides such as digoxin or digitoxin or similar medicines. Since they are markedly toxic, such plant products are generally not commercially available to the public in non-homeopathic (pharmacological) dosage forms, but the plants themselves may be obtained through cultivation or wild crafting.
(Based on references 1, 2, 5, 7, 10, and 65.)

Canadian hemp roots *(*Apocynum cannabinum, Apocynum androsaemifolium*)
Christmas rose roots *(*Helleborus niger*)
Grecian foxglove leaves *(*Digitalis lanata*)
Lily of the valley roots *(*Convallaria majalis*)
Oleander leaves *(*Nerium oleander*)
Pheasant's eye plant *(*Adonis vernalis*)

Purple foxglove leaves *(*Digitalis purpurea*)
Squill bulb leaf scales *(*Urginea maritima, Urginea indica*)
Star of Bethlehem bulbs *(*Ornithogalum umbellatum*)
Strophanthus seeds *(*Strophanthus kombe, Strophanthus hispidus*)

### Section B.2.2    Potassium Depletors

Other medicinal plants that can induce toxic effects of digitaloid glycosides, such as fibrillations, include those which cause a decrease in serum potassium levels. These incompatible plants can cause a significant loss of potassium in the stool or in the urine when used chronically or in large amounts.
(Based on references 3, 6, 10 and 65.)

**a. Laxatives**
Aloes resin *(*Aloe* spp.)
Asparagus fruit and plant (*Asparagus officinalis*)
Blue flag roots/rhizome*(*Iris versicolor*)
Buckthorn fruit *(*Rhamnus cathartica*)
Butternut bark *(*Juglans cinerea*)
Cascara sagrada bark *(*Rhamnus purshiana*)
Castor bean oil (*Ricinus communis*)
Colocynth unripe fruit pulp *(*Citrullus colocynthis*)
Frangula bark *(*Rhamnus frangula*)
Gamboge bark exudate *(*Garcinia* spp.)
Jalap roots *(*Exogonium purga*)
Leptandra root *(*Veronicastrum virginicum*)
Manna ash bark exudate (*Fraxinus ornus*)
Mayapple root *(*Podophyllum peltatum*)
Rhubarb root *(*Rheum palmatum*)
Senna leaves and pods *(*Cassia* spp.)
Wild cucumber fruit *(*Ecballium elaterium*)
Yellow dock root (*Rumex crispus*)

**b. Diuretics**
Asparagus shoots (*Asparagus officinalis*)
Buchu leaves *(*Barosma betulina*)
Celery seed (*Apium graveolens*)
Cleavers plant (*Galium aparine*)
Cocoa seeds (*Theobroma cacao*)
Corn silk (*Zea mays*)
Coffee beans *(*Caffea arabica*)

Couch grass rhizomes (*Agropyron repens*)
Goldenrod leaves and tops (*Solidago* spp.)
Gravelroot root (*Eupatorium purpureum*)
Horsetail plant *(*Equisetum* spp.)
Juniper berries *(*Juniperus* spp.)
Pareira root (*Chondodendron tomentosum*)
Parsley fruit *(*Petroselinum sativum*)
Queen Ann's lace seeds (*Daucus carota*)
Scotch broom *(*Cytisus scoparius*)
Shepherd's purse plant (*Capsella bursa-pastoris*)
Sourwood leaves (*Oxydendron arboreum*)
Tea leaves (*Camellia sinensis*)
Watermelon seeds (*Citrullus vulgaris*)

**c. Other**
Licorice root *(*Glycyrrhiza glabra*)

## *B.3   Potentiating Sedative Or Tranquilizing Medicines*

Plant products have long been used to help promote sleep, allay
anxiety, and relax muscular tension or spasms. Combining such plants
with tranquilizers and sedatives including antihistamines will further
enhance their sedative effects. This can potentially endanger the user
when the additive effect impairs cognitive, somatic, or sensory function
significantly, such as reducing alertness and reaction time when
operating a motor vehicle or working with machinery.
(Based on references 3, 5, 7, 51, and 65.)

Balm plant (*Melissa officinalis*)
Black cohosh roots/rhizome *(*Cimicifuga racemosa*)
Calendula flowers (*Calendula officinalis*)
California poppy plant (*Eschscholtzia californica*)
Catnip leaves (*Nepeta cataria*)
Chamomile, German flowers (*Matricaria recutita*)
Hops strobiles (*Humulus lupulus*)
Jamaica dogwood bark *(*Piscidia erythrina*)
Kava-kava root (*Piper methysticum*)
Lavender leaves and flowers (*Lavandula officinalis*)
Motherwort plant (*Leonurus cardiaca*)
Passion flower plant *(*Passiflora incarnata*)
Siberian ginseng (*Eleutherococcus senticosus*)
Skullcap plant (*Scutellaria laterfolia*)

St. John's wort plant (*Hypericum perforatum*)
Valerian root/rhizome *(*Valeriana officinalis*)
Wild lettuce plant (*Lactuca virosa*)
Yerba mansa root/rhizome (*Anemopsis californica*)

## B.4 Modifying Blood Sugar In Insulin-Dependent Diabetics

### Section B.4.1 Hypoglycemic Herbs

Certain plants have a well-documented ability to lower blood sugar levels through a variety of mechanisms. These are usually administered in type II diabetes (non-insulin-dependent). Insulin-dependent diabetics (type I) must monitor their blood sugar carefully to prevent hyperglycemic and hypoglycemic episodes. The combined effect of hypoglycemic herbs with insulin treatment can disrupt the means by which diabetics maintain suitable blood sugar levels and avoid insulin shock. For some plants the oral hypoglycemic activity has been confirmed for a particular extract or an identified constituent.

Some hydrocolloidal fiber sources taken in large quantities can delay gastric emptying and reduce the rate of absorption of dietary carbohydrates. (See appendix B.1.1.)

(Based on references 3, 10, 88, 89, 90, 91, 92, and 93.)

Aceitilla plant (*Bidens pilosa*)
Adiantum plant (*Adiantum capillus-veneris*)
Akee apple seeds *(*Blighia sapida*)
Banana flowers and roots (*Musa sapientum*)
Banyan stem bark *(*Ficus bengalensis*)
Barley sprouts (*Hordeum vulgare*)
Barleria plant (*Hygrophila auriculata*)
Bilberry leaves (*Vaccinium myrtillus*)
Bitter melon fruit (*Momordica charantia*)
Box thorn leaves (*Lycium barbarum*)
Bugleweed plant (*Lycopus virginicus*)
Burdock roots (*Arctium lappa*)
Cashew leaves (*Anacardium occidentale*)
Catarinita flowers (*Salpianthus arenarius*)
Coccinia roots (*Coccinia grandis*)
Copalchi root bark (*Coutarea latiflora*)
Corn silk (*Zea mays*)

Cucumber fruit (*Cucumis sativus*)
Cumin seed (*Cuminum cyminum*)
Damiana leaves (*Turnera diffusa*)
Dandelion plant (*Taraxacum officinale*)
Devil's club root bark (*Fatsia horrida*) = (*Oplopanax horridum*)
Fenugreek seeds (*Trigonella foenum-graecum*)
Fluggea seeds (*Securinega virosa*)
Garlic cloves *(*Allium sativum*)
Ginseng roots (*Panax ginseng*)
Goat's rue seeds (*Galega officinalis*)
Guarumo leaves and stem (*Cecropia obtusifolia*)
Gulancha plant (*Tinospora cordifolia*)
Gymnema leaves (*Gymnema sylvestre*)
Injerto flowers, leaves, and stem (*Psittacanthus calyculatus*)
Jambul seeds (*Syzygium jambolanum*)
Jute leaves (*Corchorus olitorius*)
Kidney bean immature pods (*Phaseolus vulgaris*)
Lagerstroemia leaves and ripe fruit (*Lagerstroemia speciosa*)
Lotus roots (*Nymphaea lotus*)
Lupin seeds (*Lupinus albus*)
Madagascar periwinkle leaves (*Catharanthus roseus*)
Mulberry leaves (*Morus* spp.)
Olive leaves (*Olea europaea*)
Onion bulbs (*Allium cepa*)
Rivea leaves (*Argyreia cuneata*)
Prickly pear stems and fruit (*Opuntia* spp.)
Sacred basil plant (*Ocimum sanctum*)
Salt bush leaves (*Atriplex halimus*)
Siberian ginseng (*Eleutherococcus senticosus*)
Solomon's seal root (*Polygonatum multiflorum*)
Spinach leaves (*Spinacea oleracea*)
Staghorn sumach leaves (*Rhus typhina*)
Stinging nettle plant (*Urtica dioica*)
Sweet broom plant (*Scoparia dulcis*)
Thorny burnet root bark (*Sarcopoterium spinosum*)
Tronadora leaves (*Tecoma stans*)
Wheat leaves (*Triticum sativum*)

## Section B.4.2 Hyperglycemic Herbs

Hyperglycemic herbs that raise blood sugar are obviously counterproductive in diabetes. In this case, aside from plants high in sugar or other carbohydrates, the known offenders are limited among commonly-used plants to a few species, mostly those containing caffeine.

(Based on references 8 and 93.)

Annato seeds (*Bixa orellana*)
Cocoa seeds (*Theobroma cacao*)
Coffee beans *(*Caffea arabica*)
Cola seed (*Cola nitida*)
Rosemary leaves (*Rosmarinus officinalis*)
Tea leaves (*Camellia sinensis*)

# Appendix C

## HERBS CONTRAINDICATED FOR MOTHERS

### C.1   During Pregnancy

The use of plants or other substances affecting normal or abnormal functions in the human body should not be used during pregnancy unless there is a known need for such agents. Indiscriminate experimentation with herbal or chemical drugs or medicines is an irresponsible act, particularly when it endangers the life, health, and future of a vulnerable and defenseless life carried in the womb. Trained and knowledgeable doctors, pharmacists, or practitioners of the healing art and science of prescribing should be consulted for information, advice, or instructions on the appropriate use of medicinal agents, most especially during pregnancy.

Pregnancy is a special time, when ordinary influences can have extraordinary consequences. Uterine contractions or significant changes in uterine tone can have disastrous effects, since carrying a baby to term necessitates stability. Alterations in uterine circulation may disrupt normal processes. Rapid system and organ growth is especially vulnerable to substances that interfere with cellular division. Abnormal hormonal influences may result in permanent developmental alterations.

Plants that have been used down through the centuries in treating women's reproductive functions have demonstrated distinctive effects on the uterus. Those that enable the onset of menstruation are known as **emmenogogues (E)**. Those that have induced miscarriages are called **abortifacients (A)**. If the use of plants causes uterine contractions, they are **uterine stimulants (US)**. Plants acting as uterine stimulants that enhance or speed labor are known as **oxytocics (O)**. All such plants may disrupt pregnancy by expelling the embryo or fetus prematurely or by partially shearing the placenta from the uterus, leading to uterine hemorrhage and/or fetal, and possibly maternal, death. Certain **uterine relaxants (UR)** that can diminish spasms may also reduce uterine tone or interfere with effective labor.

---

\* Denotes herbs in this appendix having other side effects when taken in excessive doses.

Relatively large quantities of plant substances that stimulate the uterus are usually needed to produce undesirable effects in pregnancy. Sometimes even toxic amounts must be taken. In cases where a toxic excess of irritant volatile antiseptics for the urinary tract or irritant cathartics for the intestinal tract is used, uterine stimulation may occur reflexively.

Other plants can influence normal cellular reproduction. Substances that interfere with the mother's hormonal balance or fetal genetic expression may disrupt fetal development. In the cases of gender-specific reproductive organs, plants causing **hormonal (H)** changes can alter normal expression. **Teratogens (T)** can interfere with normal development of a multiplicity of structures. **Mutagens (M)** and **genotoxins (G)** can likewise prevent normal growth. Plants with **fetotoxins (F)** endanger the very life of the developing child. In cases where these effects occur, birth defects are the unfortunate result.

In many cases portions of a plant or its extracts have been shown to have the above-mentioned effects, but in some instances only isolated chemical compounds or **components (c)** of the plant have been shown to demonstrate a particular activity. In the cases where only an isolated constituent has shown activity, the use of the crude plant part or extract is probably safe in reasonable quantities.

(Based on references 2, 3, 4, 6, 7, 10, 74, and 75)

Agave plant (*Agave americana*) E, A
Alfalfa plant (*Medicago sativa* var. *italica*) USc
Aloes exudate *(*Aloe* spp.) E, A
Amolillo roots (*Glycyrrhiza lepidota*) E; H
Angelica plant and root (*Angelica archangelica*) E
Arnica flowers *(*Arnica montana*) US
Asafetida root (*Ferula assa-foetida*) Ec, A
Ashwagandha root (*Withania somnifera*) A
Balm leaves and flowers (*Melissa officinalis*) E; H
Barberry root bark *(*Berberis vulgaris*) USc
Basil plant (*Ocymum basilicum*) E; Mc
Bearberry leaves (*Arctostaphylos uva-ursi*) O
Beet seeds, root, and leaves (*Beta vulgaris*) E, A
Betelnut seed *(*Areca catechu*) T, F
Bitter melon fruit (*Momordica charantia*) E, A
Black cohosh roots/rhizome *(*Cimicifuga racemosa*) E
Black horehound leaves and flowers (*Ballota nigra*) E
Black pepper fruit (*Piper nigrum*) A
Blazing star root *(*Aletris farinosa*) US

Bloodroot rhizome *(*Sanguinaria canadensis*) US
Buchu leaves *(*Barosma betulina*) US
Buckthorn fruit *(*Rhamnus cathartica*) US
Bugleweed leaves (*Lycopus* spp.) H
Burdock root (*Arctium lappa*) US, O
Butterbur rhizome *(*Petasites hybridus*) E; G
Buttercup plant *(*Ranunculus* spp.) USc
Calamus root *(*Acorus calamus*) E
Calendula flowers (*Calendula officinalis*) E, A
California poppy plant (*Eschscholtzia californica*) USc
Camphor tree bark *(*Cinnamomum camphora*) Ec; Fc
Cardamom seeds (*Elettaria cardamomum*) E
Cascara sagrada bark *(*Rhamnus purshiana*) US
Cassia cinnamon bark (*Cinnamomum cassia*) E, A
Catnip leaves and flowers (*Nepeta cataria*) E, A
Celandine root and plant *(*Chelidonium majus*) US
Celery root and seeds (*Apium graveolens*) E, US, A
Chamomile, German plant (*Matricaria recutita*) E
Chamomile, Roman plant (*Anthemis nobilis*) E, A
Chaste tree berries (*Vitex agnus-castus*) E
Chicory root (*Cichorium intybus*) E, A
Christmas rose plant *(*Helleborus niger*) E
Cinchona bark *(*Cinchona* spp.) US, Oc, A; T, Fc
Cinnamon bark (*Cinnamomum zeylanicum*) Ec
Coca leaves *(*Erythroxylon coca*) E; F
Coffee beans *(*Coffea arabica*) Ac; Tc
Colocynth root *(*Citrullus colocynthis*) A
Coltsfoot leaves *(*Tussilago farfara*) A
Columba root (*Jateorhiza palmata*) USc
Comfrey root *(*Symphytum officinale*) F
Cotton root bark (*Gossypium herbaceum*) E, O, A
Croton seed oil *(*Croton tiglium*) A
Dill fruit (*Anethum graveolens*) E
Dormilon plant (*Rudbeckia hirta*) E
Ergot sclerotium on rye kernerls *(*Claviceps purpura*) E, US, O, A
Fennel fruit (*Foeniculum vulgare*) E; H
Fenugreek seed (*Trigonella foenum-graecum*) E, US, A
Feverfew plant (*Tanacetum parthenium*) E
Flax seeds *(*Linum usitatissimum*) E
Frangula bark *(*Rhamnus frangula*) US
Garlic bulbs *(*Allium sativum*) E, US
Ginger rhizome (*Zingiber officinale*) A

Goldenseal root/rhizome *(*Hydrastis canadensis*) USc
Gotu kola plant (*Centella asiatica*) A
Guggul gum-resin (*Commiphora mukul*) E, A
Hemp agrimony plant *(*Eupatorium cannabinum*) E, A; F
Hibiscus flowers (*Hibiscus rosa-sinensis*) E, A
Horehound plant (*Marrubium vulgare*) E, US, A
Horse radish fresh root (*Armoracia rusticana*) A
Hyssop plant (*Hyssopus officinalis*) E, A
Inmortal root *(*Asclepias capricornu*) E, O, A
Ipecac root *(*Cephalis ipecacuanha*) USc
Jaborandi leaves *(*Pilocarpus jaborandi*) US; T
Jalap root *(*Exogonium purga*) E
Juniper berries *(*Juniperus communis*) E, US
Kava-kava root (*Piper methysticum*) UR
Khella fruit *(*Ammi visnaga*) E, US
Kousso flower *(*Brayera anthelmintica*) A
Knot grass plant (*Polygonum aviculare*) A
Lavender flowers (*Lavandula officinalis*) E
Lemon grass plant (*Cymbopogon citratus*) US
Leptandra root *(*Veronicastrum virginicum*) A; T
Licorice root *(*Glycyrrhiza glabra*) E; H
Life root plant *(*Senecio aureus*) E, O; T
Lobelia plant or seeds *(*Lobelia inflata*) UR
Lovage root (*Levisticum officinale*) E
Madder root (*Rubia tinctorum*) E; G
Ma huang plant *(*Ephedra sinica*) US
Male fern rhizome *(*Dryopteris filix-mas*) A
Mallow plant (*Malva* spp.) E
Marjoram plant (*Origanum marjorana*) E
Marsh tea plant *(*Ledum palustre*) US, A
Masterwort plant (*Heracleum lanatum*) E
Mayapple root/rhizome *(*Podophyllum peltatum*) T, Fc
Meadow saffron *(*Colchicum autumnale*) M,F
Milk thistle seed (*Silybum marianum*) E, USc
Mistletoe plant *(*Viscum album*) USc
Motherwort plant (*Leonurus cardiaca*) USc, E
Mugwort plant (*Artemisia vulgaris*) E, USc, A
Mustard seed *(*Brassica nigra*) A
Myrrh gum-resin (*Commiphora myrrha*) E, A
Nutmeg seeds *(*Myristica fragrans*) A
Opium poppy seed capsule exudate*(*Papaver somniferum*) Fc
Osha root (*Ligusticum porterii*) E, A

Papaya fruit and latex (*Carica papaya*) E, A
Pareira root (*Chondodendron tomentosum*) E
Parsley fruit *(*Petroselinum sativum*) E, USc, A
Passion flower leaves *(*Passiflora incarnata*) USc; Fc
Peach pit seeds *(*Prunus persica*) E, A; Fc
Pennyroyal plant *(*Hedeoma pulegioides*) E, A
Peony root (*Paeonia officinalis*) E
Peppermint leaves (*Mentha piperita*) E
Periwinkle plant *(*Vinca rosea*) A; T
Pine needles (*Pinus* spp.) A
Pleurisy root *(*Asclepias tuberosa*) US; H
Poison hemlock plant *(*Conium maculatum*) T
Pokeweed root *(*Phytolacca americana*) US
Poleo plant (*Mentha arvensis*) E, A
Poleo chino leaves (*Hedeoma oblongifolia*) E, A
Pomegranate root bark *(*Punica granatum*) E, US
Prickly ash bark (*Xanthoxylum americanum*) E
Pulsatilla plant *(*Anemone pulsatilla*) US
Queen Ann's lace seeds and leaves (*Daucus carota*) E, US, A
Raspberry leaves (*Rubus idaeus*) US; H
Rauwolfia root *(*Rauwolfia serpentaria*) USc, A; T
Rhubarb root *(*Rheum palmatum*) US
Rosemary leaves (*Rosmarinus officinalis*) Ec
Rue leaves and unripe fruit *(*Ruta graveolens*) E, USc, A
Saffron stigma and styles *(*Crocus sativa*) E, A
Sage leaves *(*Salvia officinalis*) E, A
Sagebrush plant (*Artemisia* spp.) E, A
Sandalwood wood (*Santalum album*) A
Sassafras bark *(*Sassafras albidum*) E
Savin tops *(*Juniperus sabina*) A
Scotch broom tops *(*Cytisus scoparius*) USc, Ac
Senega root *(*Polygala senega*) US
Senna leaves or pods *(*Cassia acutifolia*) US; G
Shepherd's purse plant (*Capsella bursa-pastoris*) E, US, A
St. John's wort plant (*Hypericum perforatum*) E, US, A
Stinging nettle plant (*Urtica* spp.) E, USc, A
Strophanthus seed *(*Strophanthus* spp.) USc
Tansy leaves *(*Tanacetum vulgare*) E, USc, A
Tobacco leaves *(*Nicotiana tabacum*) A; M, T, F
Turmeric rhizome (*Curcuma longa*) E, A
Thyme leaves *(*Thymus* spp.) E
Watercress plant (*Nasturtium officinale*) E, A

Wild angelica root (*Angelica sylvestris*) E
Wild cherry bark *(*Prunus serotina*) T, F
Wild ginger root/rhizome (*Asarum canadensis*) E, A
Wild marjoram plant (*Organum vulgare*) E, A
Wood sorrel plant (*Oxalis acetosella*) E
Wormseed seeds and plant *(*Chenopodium ambrosioides*) E, A
Wormwood tops and leaves *(*Artemisia absinthium*) E, USc, A
Yarrow plant (*Achillea millefolium*) Ec, Ac
Yellow cedar leaves *(*Thuja occidentalis*) E, Ac
Yellow jasmine plant *(*Gelsemium sempervirens*) US
Yohimbe bark *(*Pausinystalia yohimbe*) Fc

## C.2   While Breast Feeding

Some active constituents of medicinal plants are excreted in breast milk intact or as metabolites that maintain the activity of the original compounds. When this occurs it is important not to expose a breast feeding infant unnecessarily to medicinal compounds.

Certain plant components are known to produce their pharmacologic effect in the nursing child. Foremost among these is the category of compounds known as anthrones that act as **laxatives (L)**. The alkaloids caffeine and ephedrine are commonly consumed **stimulants (S)** that passes into breast milk. Some compounds act as **irritants (I)** to the digestive tract and may upset the baby's stomach and cause colic. Other components are known to be potentially disruptive to organ function or tissue growth, and nursing mothers should not risk exposure of their vulnerable infants to chemicals such as **hepatotoxic pyrrolizidine alkaloids (H)**, known **genotoxins (G)**, or other compounds potentially **toxic (T)** to small children. In addition, certain plants should be avoided while nursing that have been used as **antigalactagogues (AG)** to diminish the milk supply during the weaning process.

While the plants listed here are known to be problematic when nursing, many plants have not been adequately evaluated in this regard. Do not assume that all unlisted plants are safe to use while breast feeding.

(Based on references 2, 3, 4, 5, 6, 7, 8, 20, 24, 38, and 94.)

Aloes leaf exudate *(*Aloe* spp.) - L
Basil plant (*Ocymum basilicum*) - G
Buckthorn fruit *(*Rhamnus cathartica*) - L
Bugleweed leaves (*Lycopus* spp.) - AG

Butterbur rhizome *(*Petasites hybridus*) - H
Cascara sagrada bark *(*Rhamnus purshiana*) - L
Cinchona bark *(*Cinchona* spp.) - T
Cocoa seeds (*Theobroma cacao*) - S
Coffee beans *(*Caffea arabica*) - S
Cola seeds (*Cola nitida*) - S
Coltsfoot leaves *(*Tussilago farfara*) - H
Comfrey root and leaves *(*Symphytum officinale*) - H
Frangula bark *(*Rhamnus frangula*) - L
Hemp agrimony plant *(*Eupatorium cannabinum*) - H
Jasmin flowers (*Jasminum pubescesn*) - AG
Kava-kava root (*Piper methysticum*) - T
Life root plant *(*Senecio aureus*) - H
Madder root (*Rubia tinctorum*) - G
Ma huang plant *(*Ephedra sinica*) - S
Mate leaves (*Ilex* spp.) - S
Meadow saffron corm and seed *(*Colchicum autumnale*) - T
Prickly ash bark (*Xanthoxylum americanum*) - I
Pulsatilla plant *(*Anemone pulsatilla*) - I
Rhubarb root *(*Rheum palmatum*) - L
Sage leaves *(*Salvia officinalis*) - AG
Senna leaves and pods *(*Cassia acutifolia*) - L
Tea leaves (*Camellia sinensis*) - S
Tobacco leaves *(*Nicotiana tabacum*) - T
Wintergreen leaves *(*Gaultheria procumbens*) - T

# References

1. Brinker F. "To Health With Herbs," from *Eclectic Dispensatory of Botanical Therapeutics,* vol. I, Alstat E (comp.), Eclectic Medical Publications, Portland, Oregon, 1989
2. Brinker F. *The Toxicology of Botanical Medicines,* rev. 2nd ed., Eclectic Medical Publications, Sandy, Oregon, 1996
3. Brinker F. "Botanical Medicine Research Summaries," from *Eclectic Dispensatory of Botanical Therapeutics,* vol. II, Eclectic Medical Publications, Sandy, Oregon, 1995
4. Wichtl M (ed.). *Herbal Drugs and Phytopharmaceuticals,* CRC Press, Boca Raton, 1994
5. Felter HW, Lloyd JU. *King's American Dispensatory,* Eclectic Medical Publications, Sandy, Oregon, 1993
6. De Smet PAGM et al. (eds.). *Adverse Effects of Herbal Drugs 2,* Springer-Verlag, Berlin, 1993
7. Lust J. *The Herb Book,* Bantam Books, New York, 1974
8. Boyd JR (ed.-in-chief). *Facts and Comparisons,* J.B. Lippincott Co., St. Louis, Miss., 1985
9. Ruddiman EA. *Incompatibilities in Prescriptions,* John Wiley & Sons, Inc., New York, 1925
10. Lewis WH, Elvin-Lewis MPF. *Medical Botany,* John Wiley & Sons, New York, 1977
11. Gibelli C. "The hemostatic action of Equisetum," *Arch. intern. pharmacodynamie,* 41:419-29, 1931 (C.A. 26:6019)
12. Gutierrez RMP, Laguna GY, Walkowski A. "Diuretic Activity of Mexican Equisetum," *J. Ethnopharmacol.,* 14:269-72, 1985
13. Lepor H. "Nonoperative management of benign prostatic hyperplasia," *J. Urology,* 141:1283-9, 1989
14. Albert-Puleo M. "Fennel and anise as estrogenic agents," *J. Ethnopharmacol.,* 2:337-44, 1980
15. Albert-Puleo M. "Mythobotany, pharmacology, and chemistry of thujone-containing plants and derivatives," *Econ. Bot.,* 32:65-74, 1978
16. Brinker F. "Addendum. Potential Toxicity of Larrea tridentata," *Br. J. Phytother.,* 3:30-31, 1993
17. Blumenthal M (ed.). "German Commission E Monograph for *Echinacea purpurea* herb (Purple Cone Flower Herb)," *HerbalGram,* 30:48, 1994

18. Dulloo AG, Miller DS. "The thermogenic properties of ephedrine/methylxanthine mixtures: animal studies," *Am. J. Clin. Nutr.,* 43:388-94, 1986

19. Malchow-Moller A, Larsen S, Hey H, Stokholm KH, Juhl E, Quaade F; "Ephedrine as an anorectic: the story of the 'Elsinore pill'," *Internat. J. Obesity,* 5:183-7, 1981

20. Blumenthal M, King P. "Ma huang: anceint herb, modern medicine, regulatory dilemma," *HerbalGram,* No. 35, pp. 22-6,43,56-7, 1995

21. Tamura Y, Nishikawa T, Yamada K, Yamamoto M, Kumagai A; "Effects of Glycyrrhetinic Acid and its Derivatives on $\Delta^4$-5$\alpha$- and 5$\beta$-Reductase in Rat Liver," *Arzneim.-Forsch.,* 29:647-9, 1979

22. Singh YN. "Kava: an overview," *J. Ethnopharm.,* 37:13-45, 1992

23. Jamieson DD, Duffield PH. "Positive interaction of ethanol and kava resin in mice," *Clin. Exp. Pharmacol. Physiol.,* 17:509-14, 1990

24. Brooks S (ed.). "Botanical Toxicology," *Protocol J. Bot. Med.,* 1:147-58, 1995

25. Sigmund CJ, McNally EF. "The action of a carminative on the lower esophageal sphincter," *Gastroenterol.,* 56:13-8, 1969

26. Shader RI, Greenblatt DJ. Phenelzine and the Dream Machine - Ramblings and Reflections," *J. Clin. Psychother.,* 5:65, 1985

27. Jones BD, Runikis AM. Ínteraction of Ginseng with Phenelzine," *J. Clin. Psychopharmacol.,* 7:201-2, 1987

28. Jori A, Bianchetti A, Prestini PE, Garattini S. "Effect of eucalyptol (1,8-cineole) on the metabolism of other drugs in rats and in man," *Eur. J. Pharmacol.,* 9:362-6, 1970

29. Arch JRS, Ainsworth AT, Cawthorne MA. "Thermogenic and Anorectic Effects of Ephedrine and Congeners in Mice and Rats," *Life Sci.,* 30:1817-26, 1982

30. Astrup A, Lundsgaard C, Madsen J, Christensen NJ. "Enhanced thermogenic responsiveness during chronic ephedrine treatment in man,"*Am. J. Clin. Nutr.,* 42:83-94, 1985

31. Hogan RP III. "Hemorrhagic Diathesis Caused by Drinking an Herbal Tea," *JAMA,* 249:2679-80, 1983

32. Kempin SJ. "Warfarin resistance caused by broccoli," *New Engl. J. Med.,* 308:1229-30, 1983

33. Walker FB. "Myocardial Infarction After Diet-Induced Warfarin Resistance," *Arch. Intern. Med.,* 144:2089-90, 1984

34. Leatherdale BA, Panesar RK, Singh G, Watkins T, Bailey CJ, Bignessl AHC. "Improvement in glucose tolerance due to Momordica charantia (karela)," *Brit. Med. J.,* 282:1823-4, 1981

35. Welihinda J, Karunanayake EH, Sheriff MHR, Jayasinghe KSA. "Effect of Momordica charantia on the glucose tolerance in maturity onset diabetes," *J. Ethnopharm.*, 17:277-82, 1986

36. White RD, Swick RA, Cheeke PR. "Effects of microsomal enzyme induction on the toxicity of pyrrolizidine (*Senecio*) alkaloids," *J. Toxicol. Environ. Health,* 12:633-40, 1983

37. Brauchli J, Luthy J, Zweifel U, Schlatter C. "Pyrrolizidine alkaloids from *Symphytum officinale* L. and their percutaneous absorption in rats," *Experientia,* 38:1085-7, 1982

38. Winship KA. "Toxicity of comfrey," *Adverse Drug React. Toxicol. Tev.,* 10:47-59, 1991

39. anon., "Kelp diets can produce myxedema in iodide-sensitive individuals," *JAMA,* 233:9-10, 1975

40. Perlman BP. "Interaction between lithium salts and ispaghula husk," *Lancet,* p. 416, Feb. 17, 1990

41. Briani G, Bruttomesso D, Bilardo G, Giorato C, Duner E, Iori E, Sgnaolin E, Pedrini P, Tiengo A. "Guar-Enriched Pasta and Guar Gum in the Dietary Treatment of Type II Diabetes," *Phytother. Res.,* 1:177-9, 1987

42. Holt S, Heading RC, Carter DC, Prescott LF, Tothill P. "Effect of gel fibre on gastric emptying and absorption of glucose and paracetamol," *Lancet,* pp. 636-9, Mar. 24, 1979

43. Soci MM, Parrott EL. "Influence of Viscosity on Absorption from Nitrofurantoin Suspensions," *J. Pharm. Sci.,* 69:403-6, 1980

44. Huupponen R, Seppala P, Iisalo E. "Effect of Guar Gum, a Fibre Preparation, on Digoxin and Penicillin Absorption inMan," *Eur. J. Clin. Pharmacol.,* 26:279-81, 1984

45. Miyazaki S, Inoue H, Nadai T. "Effect of Antacids on the Dissolution Behavior of Tetracycline and Methacycline," *Chem. Pharm. Bull.,* 27:2523-7, 1977

46. Dingemanse J. "An update of recent moclobemide interaction data," *Internat. Clin. Psychopharm.,* 7:167-80, 1993

47. Dawson JK, Earnshaw SM, Graham CS. "Dangerous monoamine oxidase inhibitor interactions are still occurring in the 1990s," *J. Accident Emerg. Med.,* 12:49-51, 1995

48. Lefebvre H, Nobiet C, Moore N, Wolf LM. "Pseudo-phaeochromocytoma after multiple drug interactions involving the selective monoamine oxidase inhibitor selegiline," *Clin. Endocrin.,* 42:95-9, 1995

49. Holzl J, Demisch L, Gollnik B. "Investigations about Antidepressive and Mood Changing Effects of *Hypericum perforatum*," *Planta Med.,* 55:643, 1989

50. Sparenberg B, Demisch L, Hoelzl J. "Antidepressive constituents of St. Johnswort," *PZ Wiss.*, 6:50-4, 1993 (C.A. 119:85914z)
51. Okpanyi SN, Weischer ML. "Experimental Animal Studies of the Psychotropic Activity of a Hypericum Extract," *Arzneim.-Forsch.*, 37:10-13, 1987
52. Hendriks H, Bos R, Woerdenbag HJ, Koster AS. "Central Nervous Depressant Activity of Valerenic Acid in the Mouse," *Planta Med.*, (1):28-31, 1985
53. Tutupalli LV, Chaubal MG, Malone MH. "Saururaceae. VI. Hippocratic Screening of Anemopsis californica," *Lloydia*, 38:352-4, 1975
54. Connor J, Connor T, Marshall PB, Reid A, Turnbull MJ. "The pharmacology of Avena sativa," *J. Pharm. Pharmac.*, 27:92-98, 1975
55. Boyadzhiev T. "Sedative and hypotensive effect of preparations from the plant Calendula officinalis," *Nauchni Tr. Vissh. Med. Inst. Sofia*, 43:15-20, 1964 (C.A. 63:1114a)
56. Samochowiec L. "Pharmacological sudy of saponosides from Aralia mandshurica Rupr. et Maxim. And Calendula officinalis L.," *Herba Pol.*, 29:151-5, 1983 (C.A. 101:143586k)
57. Lee KM, Jung JS, Song DK, Krauter M, Kim YH. "Effects of Humulus lupulus Extract on the Central Nervous System in Mice," *Planta Med.*, 59(Suppl.):A691, 1993
58. Soulimani R, Fleurentin J, Mortier F, Misslin R, Derrieu G, Pelt J-M. "Neurotropic Action of the Hydroalcoholic Extract of Melissa officinalis in the Mouse," *Planta Med.*, 57:105-9, 1991
59. Wagner H, Sprinkmeyer L. "Pharmacological effect of balm spirit," *Deut. Apoth.-Ztg.*, 113:1159-66, 1973
60. Aoyagi N, Kimura R, Murata T. "Studies on Passiflora incarnata Dry Extract. I. Isolation of Maltol and Pharmacological Action of Maltol and Ethyl Maltol," *Chem. Pharm. Bull.*, 22:1008-13, 1974
61. Kasper H, Zilly W, Fassl H, Fehle F. "The effect of dietary fiber on postprandial serum digoxin concentration in man," *Am. J. Clin. Nutr.*, 32:2436-8, 1979
62. Ink SL, Hurt HD. "Nutritional Implications of Gums," *Food Technol.*, pp. 77-82, Jan., 1987
63. Rodriguez E, Towers GHN, Mitchell JC. "Biological activities of sesquiterpene lactones," *Phytochem.*, 15:1573-80, 1976
64. Rowe AH. "Camomile (Anthemis cotula) as a skin irritant," *J. Allergy*, 5:383-8, 1934
65. D'Arcy PF. "Adverse reactions and interactions with herbal medicines. Part 2 - Drug interactions," *Adverse Drug React. Toxicol. Rev.*, 12:147-62, 1993

66. Rolland A, Fleurentin J, Lanhers M-C, Younos C, Misslin R, Mortier F, Pelt JM. "Behavioural Effects of the American Traditional Plant Eschscholzia californica: Sedative and Anxiolytic Properties," *Planta Med.,* 57:212-6, 1991

67. Vincieri FF, Celli S, Mulinacci N, SperoniE. "An approach to the study of the biological activity of Eschscholtzia californica Cham.," *Pharmacol. Res. Comm.,* 20(Suppl. V):41-4, 1988

68. Ying J, Guoqing L, Junru M, Xie L, Wu H. "Pharmacological studies on methyleugenol," *Yaoxue Xuebao,* 17:87092, 1982 (C.A. 96:192951n)

69. Engelbrecht JA, Long JP, Nichols DE, Barfknecht CF. "Pharmacologic evalution of 3,4-dimethoxyphenylpropenes and 3,4-dimethoxyphenylpropanediols," *Arch. Int. Pharmacodyn. Ther.,* 199:226-44, 1972 (C.A. 78:11566a)

70. Fluck AAJ, Mitchell W, Perry HM. "Composition of buchu leaf oil," *J. Sci. Food Agric.,* 12:290-2, 1961

71. Kaiser R, Schudel P. "Analysis of Buchu Leaf Oil," *J. Agric. Food Chem.,* 23:943-50, 1975

72. Costello CH, Butler CL. "The Estrogenic and Uterine-Stimulating Activity of Asclepias tuberosa. A Preliminary Investigation," *J. Am. Pharm. Assoc.,* 39: 233-7, 1950

73. Sinha A, Rao AR. "Embryotoxicity of betel nuts in mice," *Toxicol.,* 37:315-26, 1985

74. Farnsworth NR, Bingel AS, Cordell GA, Crane FA, Fong HHS. "Potential Value of Plants as Sources of New Antifertility Agents I," *J. Pharm. Sci.,* 64:535-98, 1975

75. Conway GA, Slocumb JC. "Plants used as abortifacients and emmenagogues by Spanish New Mexicans," *J. Ethnopharm.,* 1:241-61, 1979

76. Holmberg G, Gershow S. "Autonomic and Psychic Effects of Yohimbine Hydrochloride," *Psychopharm.,* 2:93-106, 1961

77. DeSmet PAGM, Smeets OSNM. "Potential risks of health food products containing yohimbe extracts," *Br. Med. J.,* 309:958, 1994

78. Sandler B, Aronson P. "Yohimbine-induced cutaneous drug eruption, progressive renal failure, and lupus-like syndrome," *Urology,* 41:343-5, 1993

79. Ingram CG. "Some pharmacologic actions of yohimbine and chlorpromazine in man," *Clin. Pharmacol. Therap.,* 3:345-52, 1962

80. Riley AJ. "Yohimbine in the treatment of erectile disorder," *Br. J. Clin. Pract.,* 48:133-6, 1994

81. Ferguson T. *The Smoker's Book of Health,* G.P. Putnam's Sons, New York, 1987

82. Tunnerhoff FK, Schwabe HK. "Studies in Human Beings and Animals on the Influence of Echinacea Extracts on the Formation of Connective Tissue following the Implantation of Fibrin," *Arznein.-Forsch.*, 6:330-4, 1956

83. Bodinet C, Williigmann I, Beuscher N. "Host-Resistance Increasing Activity of Root Extracts from Echinacea Species," *Planta Med.*, 59(Suppl.):A672, 1993

84. Palasciano G, Portincasa P, Palmieri V, Ciani D, Vendemiale G, Altomare E. "The Effect of Silymarin on Plasma Levels of Malon-Dialdehyde in Patients Receiving Long-Term Treatment with Psychotropic Drugs," *Curr. Ther. Res.*, 55:537-45, 1994

85. Leonforte JF, "Contact dermatitis from Larrea (creosote bush)," *J. Am. Acad. Dermatol.*, 14(2, pt.1):202-7, 1986

86. Shasky DR, "Contact dermatitis from Larrea tridentata (creosote bush)," *J. Am Acad. Dermatol.*, 15(2, pt. 1):302, 1986

87. Kleinhenz ME, Ellner JJ, Spagnuolo PJ, Daniel TM. "Suppression of Lymphocyte Responses by Tuberculous Plasma and Mycobacterial Arabinogalactan," *J. Clin. Invest.*, 68:153-621 1981

88. Perez G. RM, Ocegueda Z. A, Munoz L. JL, Avila A. JG, Morrow WW. "A Study of the Hypoglucemic Effect of Some Mexican Plants," *J. Ethnopharm.*, 12:253-62, 1980

89. Bever BO, Zahnd GR. "Plants with Oral Hypoglycaemic Action," *Quart. J. Crude Drug Res.*, 17:139-96, 1979

90. Farnsworth NR, Segelman AB. "Hypoglycemic Plants," *Tile Till*, 57:52-6, 1971

91. Roman-Ramos R, Flores-Saenz JL, Alarcon-Aguilar FJ. "Anti-hyperglycemic effect of some edible plants," *J. Ethnopharm.*, 48:25-32, 1995

92. Gonzalex M, Zarzuelo A, Gamez MJ, Utrilla MP, Jimenez J, Osuna I. "Hypoglycemic Activity of Olive Leaf," *Planta Med.*, 58:513-5, 1992

93. Al-Hader AA, Hasan ZA, Aqel MB. "Hyperglycemic and insulin release inhibitory effects of *Rosmarinum officinalis*," *J. Ethnopharm.*, 43:217-21, 1994

94. Abraham M, Sarada Devi N, Sheela R. "Inhibiting effect of jasmine flowers on lactation," *Indian J. Med. Res.*, 69:88-92, 1979

95. Linde K, Ramirez G, Mulrow CD, Pauls A, Weidenhammer W, Melchart D. "St. John's wort for depression - an overview and meta-analysis of randomised clinical trials," *Br. Med. J.*, 313:253-8, 1996

# Index

## A

abdominal pain, 29, 33, 49, 77, 81
abendlandischer lebensbaum, 91
abortifacients, 107
abraded surfaces, 48
absinthe, 90
ACACIA, 17, 99
*Acacia catechu*, 100
*Acacia senegal*, 17, 99
*Acanthopanax senticosus*, 82
Aceitilla, 104
acetaminophen, 66, 84, 86
ache des marais, 36
achicoria amarga, 38
achilee, 90
*Achillea millefolium*, 90, 96, 112
acibar, 18
acore vrai, 31
acoro aromatico, 31
*Acorus calamus*, 31, 109
actee a grappes, 24
Adiantum, 104
*Adiantum capillus-veneris*, 104
*Adonis*, 18, 29, 33, 34, 49, 77, 81
*Adonis vernalis*, 101
*Aesculus hippocastanum*, 54
Africa pepper, 35
Agar, 99
Agave, 108
*Agave americana*, 108
agneau chaste, 38
agripaume, 67
*Agropyron repens*, 103
ague grass, 26
ague tree, 79
agueweed, 27
**AIDS**, 45

ail, 50
ajenjo, 90
Akee apple, 104
ala, 46
alashi, 48
albahaca, 22
alcohol, 17, 58
alcoholism, 86
Alder, 100
alder buckthorn, 49
alder dogwood, 49
*Aletris farinosa*, 26, 108
Alexandrian senna, 80
Alexandriner-senna, 80
ALFALFA, 17, 108
Alginate, 99
alkaloids, 69, **100**
allergic hypersensitivity, 19, 20, 25, 26, 27, 34, 38, 39, 40, 44, 46, 66, 70, 73, 74, 90, 91
all-heal, 67, 87
*Allium cepa*, 105
*Allium sativum*, 50, 105, 109
*Alnus* spp., 100
Aloe, 99
*Aloe* spp., 18, 102, 108, 112
*Aloe vera*, 99
ALOES, 18, 102, 108, 112
*Althaea officinalis*, 64, 100
Alum, 100
amapola amarilla, 31
amapola de California, 31
amber, 82
**amebic dysentery**, 39
American indigo, 88
American mandrake, 65
American pennyroyal, 72
American wormseed, 89
Amerikanischer faulbaum, 32
Amerikanisches wanzenkraut, 24
**amiloride**, 60
**aminopyrine**, 46
*Ammi visnaga*, 58, 97, 110
**amobarbital**, 86, 92
Amolillo, 108
*Amorphophallus konjac*, 99

## FRANCIS BRINKER, N.D.

Francis Brinker, N.D., is a 1981 graduate of the National College of Naturopathic Medicine in Portland, Oregon. In addition, he completed the two year Postgraduate Studies Program in Botanical Medicine and taught Botanical Medicine until 1985.

Dr. Brinker's undergraduate work includes a Bachelor of Science Degree in Human Biology from Kansas Newman College and a Bachelor of Arts Degree in Biology from the University of Kansas, Phi Beta Kappa.

He is currently an instructor at the Southwest College of Naturopathic Medicine and Health Sciences and a researcher of historic, scientific and medical literature.

In addition to numerous articles published in European and U.S. professional journals, Dr. Brinker is author of *The Eclectic Dispensatory of Botanical Therapeutics, Vol. II,* and a major contributor to *The Eclectic Dispensatory of Botanical Therapeutics, Vol. I.* His work, *The Toxicology of Botanical Medicine,* is available through Eclectic Medical Publications and is recognized as the finest study of medicinal plant toxicology currently available.

Books by Francis Brinker, N.D.

The Toxicology of Botanical Medicines
The Eclectic Dispensatory of Botanical Therapeutics, Vol. II
Formulas For Healthful Living